AUTISM:

BECOMING A

PROFESSIONAL

PARENT

—·—

(1) EXPLORING THE SENSORY WORLD OF AUTISM

OLGA BOGDASHINA

 Life & Learn

ISBN: 978-1-7398181-0-4

British Library Cataloguing-in-Publication data

A catalogue record for this book is available from the British Library

Publications in other languages

First published in Romanian in 2018: "Cum devenim părinţi profesionişti (1) Explorând lumea senzorială a autismului" Iaşi; © Octombrie 2018; ISBN 978-606-13-4601-1

In Macedonian: "Аутизам: Да се биде професионален родител: (1) Истражување на сензорниот свет на аутизмот" Арс Ламина, Скопје © 2019, Арс Ламина; ISBN 978-608-259-356-2

In Russian: «Аутизм: Стать профессиональным родителем: (1) Изучение сенсорного мира аутизма» Международный Институт Аутизма, Красноярский гос. пед. университет, © 2019, Международный Институт Аутизма

In Italian: "Autismo: Diventare un genitore professionista (1) Esplorando il mondo sensoriale dell'autismo", Associazione l'Ortica, Milano; © 2019, Associazione l'Ortica, Milano; ISBN 978-88-944460-0-5

In Hungarian: Cím: Hogyan legyek legjobb szülő (1). Az autizmus érzékelésvilágának felfedezése Szerző; Kiadó: Geobook Hungary © 2021, Geobook Hungary Kiadó, ISBN: 9786155015618

First published in English in 2022 by Life & Learn

 Life & Learn

To my children, Alyosha and Olesya

CONTENTS

ACKNOWLEDGMENTS

Like all my books, this one would not have been written if it were not for my children (who are young adults now) – Alyosha and Olesya. It's Alyosha and Olesya who have helped me develop not only into an '(autism) professional parent' but also learn about my Self. Without them, I wouldn't have become the 'me' I am now.

The largest debt of gratitude goes to my first autistic students: Vita, Pavlik, Dima and Sasha, and the autistic individuals who are willing to share their experiences and ideas in order to help us all learn about the diversity of human perception of the world.

My everlasting gratitude goes to an extraordinary autistic artist, Peter Myers, who's provided me with his drawings to illustrate autistic creativity, and Ian Wilson, a brilliant artist working with adults with autism, who kindly drew the picture of the Weak Central Coherence (WCC) for this book and designed the icons for the sections.

My special thanks are due to the parents and their children who gave me permission to use their drawings in this book, and those who share their concerns and ideas of bringing up their autistic children.

A big thank you to Debby Elley, journalist and mum with autism, co-editor of *Aukids* (a fun, yet educational magazine that offers a lot of support to parents who are learning about autism in a very innovative way through its advice columns, expert opinions and other informative articles). It was Debby (though she might not know it) who gave me the idea for this book, when she sent me an invitation to contribute to the magazine.

And of course, thanks are also due to Nigel, Lucy and Peter, whose emotional support throughout the project was invaluable.

— · —

INTRODUCTION

M y life can be divided into two distinct and very different lives – BA (Before Alyosha was born) and AA (After Alyosha was born in 1988).

The final stages of BA: MEd (Teaching Methods; foreign languages), MPhil (Psychology), PhD (Linguistics); Professor, Head of the Linguistics Department in the Pedagogical University of Foreign Languages (Gorlovka, Ukraine).

The initial stage of AA: Lost and confused as my autistic son was considered "unteachable, unmanageable and hopeless" and was offered a placement in a special institution for severely mentally retarded children outside the town.

Not much (if anything) was known about autism in Ukraine (where I happened to live at that time), so I re-directed my research skills from linguistics to autism. Starting from scratch and lacking any professional guidance was a blessing in disguise: my ignorance to 'common knowledge' about autism meant that I wasn't restricted by the well-known (in the West) influential theoretical constructs but rather, I had an advantage

1

to establish a balanced view of different schools in autism research. Comparing British and American theories and approaches and getting experience of working with 'unteachable' children in my school (set up in 1994 – for my son and other 'ineducable and unmanageable' children who were denied the state education) provided me with a wonderful opportunity to start my first research project in sensory perceptual differences in autistic children.

The reason I considered sensory issues as more important than any triadic[1] part of the condition was again... my ignorance – at the time I didn't know that it was not essential for diagnosis. For me, it was obvious – these children's 'abnormal' or 'bizarre' reactions to sensory stimuli indicated that their perception of the world was different; and these differences in sensory perception impact not only on behaviours but also lead to atypical cognitive, emotional, language, communication and social development.

Both life journeys contain learning curves, successes and failures but the second one differs in one important aspect – not only have I learnt about autism and my son's worldview, I've actually started to understand my Self, who/what I really am (and what an idiot I was in my 'BA life'). Memory flashbacks make me feel embarrassed when I suddenly 'see' for the first time how other people looked at my behaviour in some situations. Now I realise why I myself, have never even considered anything being wrong – I was living in an 'autistic environment' from the day I was born [my father (a mathematician) and my elder brother (a historian) would be diagnosed with Asperger syndrome today], so everything was 'normal'. I recognise my family's traits – though hugely exaggerated – in my son.

By the time I came to the UK to write my dissertation on the topic of sensory perception in autism I had gathered a huge amount of theoretical and practical evidence. This first project resulted in my first book in English – *Sensory Perceptual Issues in Autism and Asperger Syndrome: Different Sensory Experiences – Different Perceptual Worlds*[2].

The research has shown that 'sensory symptoms' can be noticed very early in life, long before the social interaction and communication difficulties. There is a continuum of sensory perceptual problems/differences in autism[3]. Some children have severe sensory distortions while others may experience only mild but nevertheless confusing sensory problems. However, there is a very important point to take into account – not all the differences in perception are dysfunctional and sensory processing differences are not necessarily problems/difficulties. Some may be interpreted as strengths or even superabilities that can become 'dysfunctional' if not recognised and accommodated by the outside world.

Let us take two examples:
· Some difficulties are caused by environmental factors. If a child is hypersensitive to fluorescent lights, his/her 'dysfunction' will be noticeable only in rooms with fluorescent lighting. If it is accommodated, for example, the child wears special sunglasses, this particular 'dysfunction' will disappear.
· Autistic individuals have some perceptual abilities that are superior to non-autistic people. The problem is,

3

non-autistic people cannot appreciate them because they do not know these abilities exist! Imagine that you are unable to see the colour red - how could you appreciate the beauty of red roses? If the majority cannot see it, the ability to enjoy the 'redness' becomes useless and... dysfunctional.

My son is now 34. From a non-verbal autistic child (he didn't talk till he was seven), he has developed into a bilingual autistic young man. He goes to a day centre four times a week. And although he cannot live independently yet and needs someone to be with him, we never say never!

* * * * *

This is the first of a series of small books [*Autism: Becoming a Professional Parent (1)*] in which I share what I've learned (and continue to learn) about autism. The idea's come from my presentations at conferences and trainings at schools and residential settings – where I often illustrate the theoretical points with examples from my experience of living and working with autistic children, teenagers and adults; and from the blog (I was a columnist in 'Aukids').

The first part of this series (*Exploring the Sensory World of Autism*) covers a range of sensory perceptual issues and provides ideas and tips how to help the child, which will inspire and inform those who live and/or work with autistic children. However, this is especially aimed for parents with autistic children, and will guide them through the ins- and outs of not just living with – but flourishing – together with their autistic children.

There are 12 chapters in the book. Each chapter is in two parts:

1. A personal story, illustrating one or two sensory problems that are common in autism
2. Information and research related to the topic raised in the first part. It is subdivided into four sections:

 Notes in the Margin: explanation of the phenomena and additional information of the issue introduced in the first part

 There is always a BUT: what else should be taken into account

 Tips (Do's and Don'ts): Practical advice and tips (what can be done to help the child / what should be avoided)

 Pause for Thought: Another short personal story or an essay to make the reader reflect on their own experiences.

At the end of the book, you can find Notes (with additional information and references) and Glossary for some terms used in the book (the words explained in the glossary are marked with an asterisk (*))

1

TWO LIVES FOR THE PRICE OF ONE

I t's a strange feeling to have two lives in one lifetime. But that is exactly what happened to me. I even know the date of my second 'conception' – 14 July 1988. No, for me it wasn't an anniversary of the French Revolution. This was the day when my son was born.

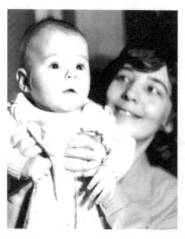

The baby who's changed the trajectory of my life

As far as I remembered I'd always wanted to be a mum. At the time, I was Professor and the head of the Linguistics department at Gorlovka University, Eastern Ukraine. If everything had happened the way I thought it would, I could have added the title of 'mum' to my professional MA, MSc and Ph.D. qualifications, while continuing to teach my students amazing facts about the history of the English language, complexities of theoretical grammar, as well as English and American literature.

However, my dream-life lasted only for about 12 months. During this time, I spent as much time with my baby as I could, doing everything according to the book and enjoying every minute of being responsible for this perfect baby. Though born three weeks premature and having had feeding problems during the first three months, Alyosha *was* perfect. The most obvious feature that triggered so many flattering comments from strangers when I proudly took him for his daily walks in the park, and from friends and relatives when they came to visit was his angelic appearance. He was (and is) very good-looking.

The perfection was not limited only to his good looks. It shone through his quiet disposition and contentment with his life. He was smiling most of the time and I tried to understand what made him so happy when nobody was around. As a bonus, Alyosha seemed unusually intelligent for his age. His eyes were so deep and wise, more suitable for a middle-aged philosopher than a tiny infant. When my little professor looked at me, he seemed to penetrate inside my very soul.

Most of the time when awake, Alyosha was content with his own company and would sit in his cot for hours, surrounded with his toys. He wouldn't play with them, but rather tap or scratch them with his fingers or spin the wheels of a toy car for what seemed to be eternity. What my friends saw as good fortune ('Your son is a perfect baby. You are so lucky!'), however, was beginning to worry me. He didn't make any demands for my attention and appeared uninterested when I offered it. Was he really just a perfect baby? No, something was definitely wrong, and soon it was impossible not to notice this 'something'.

In a matter of weeks, Alyosha changed from a perfect baby into a little monster. He became hyperactive, constantly on the move, jumping up and down, whirling himself like a top, or running in circles clutching his favourite toy. At night, he stubbornly refused to go to bed without me. As a baby, he used to lie in his pram for hours, never demanding any attention from me. As he grew, if I wasn't by his side, singing, he would scream at the top of his voice until I returned. My 'solo-concerts' lasted for hours. Any attempt to move away was met with not very musical screams from my audience.

At the age of two and a half years, Alyosha was referred to a 'psychiatric consultation board' (by the doctor who had originally told me my son didn't talk because he was 'just lazy' and his development was 'normal'. She didn't reveal the reason that made her change her mind). The result of this consultation was shocking: the board dubbed Alyosha 'unteachable', 'unmanageable' and – what infuriated me most – 'hopeless'. My boy was offered a placement in a special institution for 'ineducable children'. Did these 'specialists' expect me to accept their 'verdict'? My conclusion (emotions aside) was that they didn't have a clue what they were talking about, so it was up to me to learn as much as I could about my son's condition and find out how I can help him. The problem was, however, I didn't know *what* it was I had to learn about.

In the beginning was the word

One day, by pure chance, an American psychiatrist saw my son and when I asked for his opinion, it was the first time I heard the word – AUTISM. Learning that my boy was autistic brought... relief. I've never thought of autism as 'good' or 'bad'. The word 'autism' had no emotional connotations for me – it was neutral – the condition I had to research in order to find ways to help my son. I knew from the start that autism was for life but it didn't bother me. The main thing was that I wasn't blind to what was going on anymore. The next step was to educate myself to become powerful enough to change the situation to my son's advantage. From that day onwards, I redirected my research skills from linguistics to autism and started my long journey of learning and discovery.

During the day, I continued to supervise the staff of my department and to give lectures and seminars to my students introducing them to the world of linguistics. It was at night when I nurtured my real interest – the world of autism. It quickly became my obsession. Although degrees in linguistics, psychology and education did help in my research quest, the more I learned, the more I realised how little I knew. My long journey as a 'permanent student' in autism started in earnest and is still continuing until this day.

* * * * *

Notes in the margin – Possible scenarios of early development

Autism is rarely (if ever) detected from birth. From my work with parents of autistic children, I've drawn several possible scenarios of their experiences with their offspring who would be diagnosed with autism later:

- A perfect baby:
o may sleep through the night and take scheduled naps during the day
o rarely cries, seeming content with everything
o coos, smiles
o reaches milestones in time
o typically evokes this response from relatives and friends – 'You are so lucky. He/she is a perfect baby.'

- A 'handful' baby:
o does not sleep much
o has feeding problems
o has ear infection after ear infection
o cannot be left alone for a minute
o screams without any apparent reason
o is always 'on the go'.
- A combination of these: for example, a child may start as a 'perfect' baby and develop into a 'handful' one. [My son's case]

There's always a BUT - Early signs that can be overlooked

Some early signs of autism may be overlooked[1]:
- a fascination with lights, sounds, smells, textures, body movements,
- happy when left alone,
- doesn't like to be held,
- rocking,
- low muscle tone (in infancy),
- spinning, tapping/scratching objects,
- excessive blinking,
- flapping arms or hands,
- sniffing objects, people,
- playing with parts of toys (e.g., a wheel of a car),
- lining up objects,
- doesn't like it when his toys have been touched or rearranged,
- screaming when his hair is washed, or his nails are cut,
- hair once soft, may become wiry and coarse,
- unusual body postures,
- walking on tip-toes,
- running in circles,
- drops things,
- motor-coordination problems,
- difficulties coordinating arm and leg movement, e.g., not moving arms when walking/running,
- poor gross and fine motor skills[4]

- refusing to use his hands, e.g., at meal-times refuses to hold a spoon/fork,
- unusual food preferences,
- limited diet,
- no recognition of familiar adults when they change their clothes, hair style,
- no reaction to loud sound/ his or her name (suspected deafness, but may be alert when the slightest noise is heard, for example, opening a box of biscuits)
- may start talking and then:
o loses the words
o idiosyncratic language development

[1] However, just because a child shows *some of these symptoms*, it doesn't necessarily mean a diagnosis of autism.

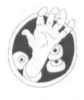 ## Do's and Don'ts

When you learn that your child has autism:
- Feeling pity for yourself? No problem: take your time – cry, grieve, consider how unfair the world is, or whatever you want to grieve about – but not too long. Then look at your baby (the age of the 'baby' doesn't matter) – it is your precious child who needs your love, your understanding and your help.
- Remember, you're not alone and yours is not the only family with an autistic child. Many others are in the same boat. Find them. They've been there, done that, and will be happy to share their experiences with you and provide you with valuable tips and advice.

-      The strategies the parents use to reconsider their attitudes and find the way to accept the challenge are as different as the backgrounds and circumstances of the families. Let go all your dreams (expectations and assumptions) of what you wanted your child to be. You have the child you have. Here and now. Your child has autism. You have to deal with it. Autism is NOT the end of the world/ God's punishment/ a catastrophe, etc.

-      But don't make a mistake idealising the condition, either – it won't help you or your child if you take a stance 'autism is beautiful and we shouldn't do anything about it'. In fact, the worst thing you can do is to do nothing. Autism (like non-autism) is neither good nor bad. Yes, it involves a lot of changes in the life of the family – teaching the child and learning from the child the ways to communicate that are very different from our conventional understanding of communication, but very soon the understanding of these new world-views and interactions will bring *normality* into the family life.

When asked what it was like to live with an autistic brother, my daughter (15 years old at the time) replied: "What do you mean 'what's it like? It's normal!"

-      Educate yourself. There is a lot of information available now. Read as much as you can, ask questions, discuss the issues you worry about with specialists and other parents. Be aware, however, that the spectral character of autism means that not everything you read will apply to your child, so find the information that is useful for your circumstances.

-      The child is developing, so what's right for him/her today can be useless/wrong tomorrow.

-     Don't expect your learning and finding solutions to all the challenges to be easy - new answers will bring more questions. Learning about autism never stops. (I found consolation in the principle I formulated in the very beginning: Whatever autism is, it is never boring.)
-     Not everything will go smoothly. You will make mistakes (and learn from them). Comments (and stares) from onlookers did (and do) hurt. You have to develop a really thick skin or fight back (respond), or both.

 ## Pause for Thought – Difficult Children - Difficult Parents

Autism is, probably, the most difficult of all disabilities (or conditions) to cope with. Of course, it would be wrong to define disabilities as 'better' or 'worse', but it is justifiable to assume that autism does bring a great strain in families, incomparable to other disorders.

There are several reasons for this. Firstly, very often autism is difficult to identify; it is in a way 'invisible'. There is no evidence of any disability in the child's appearance, in contrast, for instance, to children with cerebral palsy, Down syndrome, or physical impairments. Hence, the child's often 'bizarre' behaviour is misunderstood and misinterpreted ('spoilt, naughty child') and parents are under constant stress for being blamed for their inability to discipline their offspring.

Secondly, in addition to the negative attitude from the outside, parents often feel rejected by their own child, creating a feeling of uselessness and unreturned love.

And thirdly, it is a great physical and emotional strain to raise a child who can go without any sleep for more than 20 hours, who doesn't eat food prepared for him/her, who might be aggressive and get into a meltdown out of the blue – in short, a child who needs 24-hour supervision, each day, every day.

It's not only the children who develop, their parents develop as well. There are several possible scenarios of parents' development. The time between diagnosis and acceptance can be very long and very painful, a period during which parents go through several stages:

1. Denial: They don't want to believe that their beautiful, beloved son or daughter has a problem. Sometimes they do feel that something is wrong with their child. At other times, however, they persuade themselves that all is well, that their child is developing normally. (He passed his major milestones at the usual ages, didn't he? She is so good at switching on the TV or finding the video she wants, isn't she?) They find their situation hard to accept, and very often get offended when friends or relatives suggest that they consult a doctor. To stay at this stage too long is very dangerous, as the sooner the diagnosis is made and the right support is introduced, the better chances the child has for the future.

2. Shock: The reality of having a child with autism often causes shock, which can be then followed by:

3. Helplessness: At this stage, parents are emotionally paralysed, unable to do anything. At first, they feel helpless because they don't know much about autism and what they are to do. Paradoxically, the more the parents learn about the condition, the more confused and helpless they sometimes feel. Very often, they think that they are the only family in the world to have a child like this, that nobody else can understand their problems. (To know that there are many others in the same situation brings a great relief and desire to seek help.)

4. Guilt: Parents may feel guilt, and question if they are to blame for their child's disability. This is the stage when families either get stronger, uniting their efforts to help the child, or split up because the parents blame each other or each other's relatives in having 'the wrong gene'. Along with guilt often comes shame. Some parents (especially, in certain cultures) become ashamed of their child, not wanting to take him out in public, or reluctant to talk about him with their friends as if he didn't exist, etc. They view the emotional pain they experience as punishment for something they have done in the past. Fortunately, most parents move through this issue, but are met with an equally challenging set of emotions.

5. Anger: Parents then start to question their new situation, 'Why our child? What did we do wrong? Why do other parents drink, smoke and have normal children and we don't?' Sometimes, subconsciously, the parents feel pity for themselves. This is another dangerous stage to get stuck in, as parents tend to put their energy into blaming everybody and everything for their misfortune, rather than seeking help.

It is necessary to note that some parents miss one or two stages, and some stay on certain stages longer than others. After having gone through all these emotional swings, the parents approach the point with several paths to follow. The choice is very individual and depends on personal factors. Whatever road they choose, the most important thing to arrive at is acceptance.

6. Acceptance: The parents love their child for who he/she is and for the very differences that make the child unique. Another important step is to stop feeling pity for themselves and start to enjoy the company of the child. As a result, the family is happy and united in their efforts to improve the quality of the child's and the whole family's life. They become proud of their child's progress. Even the smallest signs of improvement (he buttoned his shirt, she managed to put on her socks, he answered 'yes' to the question) are seen as a triumph and victory for the whole family in their continual quest to understand their child and make him happy. The parents do not feel ashamed of their child and take him everywhere, trying to involve him in all their activities as much as possible, ignoring the stares of ill-informed people. They learn to love their child not despite the child's differences but because of them.

A very good tool to help, I think, is a good sense of humour! It can often transform a seemingly devastating situation into an amusing story to share with friends and relatives. As an example, when my son was eight and a half, there was a reception for some Ukrainian officials at the Town Hall in Barnsley where I was interpreting. My autistic son was in the same room sitting near the door with one of my friends. After the official part of the reception, an invitation to have a drink followed. At that briefest moment of complete silence when everybody turned to go to the tables, my boy said very loudly: 'But first, everybody to the toilet!' Everyone roared with laughter. Yes, I was embarrassed, but so what? It happened, and now I cannot help smiling when I remember this episode!

What is interesting is that difficult children often produce difficult parents. Perhaps it comes from our deep desire to improve our child's quality of life. (I, myself am the mother of an autistic child, and I have to confess... I too, can be difficult.)

Nevertheless, I have to also admit – I do admire the difficult parents who make the lives of their children easier.

2

—.—

AFTER THE WILDERNESS, A SENSORY JOURNEY BEGINS

L iving with my son and getting experience of working with 'unteachable' children in my school provided me with a wonderful opportunity to become an anthropologist studying a very different culture and learning to identify a very unconventional worldview. Every day more ideas jumped out, some were good, others – useless, and plenty – in-between, but the process of navigating a 'parallel world' of autistic children was fascinating in itself: taking wrong turns, getting back to the junction and starting again. Reflecting on all the experiences I had at the time, the 'I wish I had known...' thought often comes up. In a couple of months, I got a draft of the 'roadmap' and started serious research of differences in sensory perception of 'my children' that helped to see their ways to interpret (and react to) a hostile environment (which we call our 'normal' world) around them.

These days, sensory issues in autism are widely recognised. In 2013, they were officially included into the diagnostic criteria of autism – DSM-V (Diagnostic and Statistical Manual of mental Disorders, Fifth Edition); and hundreds of research papers and books on the subject of sensory perception have been published. At the time, though, nobody took me seriously.

I wish I had known...

In the beginning I made a mistake, which is quite common even now, in focussing on sensory sensitivities as the main problem (i.e., being over-sensitive, otherwise known as hypersensitive or under-sensitive, otherwise known as hyposensitive). I recognised these in my son and in the children I worked with. However, it soon became clear that these problems were actually secondary, caused by some other sensory phenomena.

It is hard to imagine that their senses work differently – They are not blind or deaf, are they? So they must perceive (see, hear, smell, etc.) the same way we do. Right?

Wrong!

Sometimes autistic children do behave as if they were blind or deaf: some touch and smell things to identify them; others tap objects to produce the sound and recognise what it is, because their visual recognition is unreliable, or they touch furniture, walls and things to figure out where the boundaries are in their environment.

Alyosha used to touch and smell objects or food to check his visual perception of them. Sometimes he shut down his vision completely and used his ears, or nose to 'see' his environment. He recognised the objects by the sounds they produced much better than their visual images. The disadvantage of this 'auditory seeing' was that when his hearing became overloaded and couldn't cope with auditory and 'visual' information, it either became hypersensitive (and painful) or shut down altogether. Then he found his 'world' unusually quiet (*the spoon has grown quiet*) and dangerous. It often led to panic attacks and outbursts.

Alyosha also had difficulty sleeping (he slept for not more than 3-4 hours at night) because 'sound images' around him made it hard for the boy to relax. All these experiences caused anxiety, stress and what we call 'challenging behaviours'.

One sense is never enough for autistic children to make sense of their environment. The matter is, if one or several senses are unreliable (hypersensitive, etc.) the child might use the sensory channel that he can trust – to make sense of the surroundings. For instance, in the case of visual problems, they use their ears, nose, tongue or hand to 'see': the child can tap objects to produce the sound and recognise what it is, because his visual recognition can be fragmented and meaningless. Or if there are proprioceptive problems, the child watches his feet while walking, or his hands while doing something. Vestibular difficulties can be suspected if the child avoids climbing, jumping, walking on uneven ground, or the opposite – excessive jumping, swinging, spinning.

A typical situation: a little girl with autism smells someone who's just entered the room. Her carer will no doubt think of the social situation first and foremost and tell her not to do it, it's not nice. No doubt, it's not nice. But what if the sense of smell is the most reliable sense that the child uses to get information about the world, recognise things and people? Isn't it more logical to address the child's visual/ auditory/ tactile, etc. problems first instead of shutting down the girl's only reliable channel to get the information through?

My son used to smell everything and anything. I'm very grateful to the autistic author Donna Williams who, many years ago, advised me to check his visual sensitivities. Since he started wearing his tinted glasses, he stopped using his nose to 'see' the world, his hearing seemed to 'normalise' (though it is still very acute, it doesn't hurt) and he sleeps better at night!

To many young children with autism, the senses of touch and smell are more reliable than vision or hearing. It's therefore important to let the children use whichever sense they prefer to 'check' their perception. With appropriate treatment and environmental adjustments to decrease hypersensitivities and perceptual distortions, they gradually start relying on other senses and use eyes to see, ears to listen, etc.

* * * * *

 ## Notes in the Margin – Seven Senses

Traditionally we distinguish seven senses: vision*, hearing*, vestibular system*, olfaction* (sense of smell), gustation* (sense of taste), tactility* and proprioception*

(body awareness), including interoception* (sensitivity to stimuli originating inside the body). We do not think about any other ways to perceive the world that seem to be available to (at least, some) autistic individuals.

There's always a BUT – More Senses

However, some researchers consider more senses, for instance, Guy Murchie[5] examined 32 senses, which he divided into 5 categories (the radiation senses, the feeling senses, the chemical senses, the mental senses, and the spiritual senses). There have been reports that some autistic individuals can be sensitive to radio waves. Quite a few people reveal that they can hear radio programmes when the radio is switched off but still plugged in. These cases are not that rare: for example, my friend, a 60-year-old woman with Asperger syndrome has to unplug all the electric appliances in her flat before going to bed, otherwise she would be unable to screen out the radio programmes from the switched off transistor and buzzing sounds from a (switched off yet plugged in) microwave oven, for example, which at night is very 'audible and annoying'.

Do's and Dont's

Observe how the child reacts to the surroundings. Remember, his reactions and actions are rational and logical. And he's doing his best to

23

function (or even to survive) in the environment he can't (physically) tolerate.

There is no single strategy for all autistic children as each of them exhibits a very individual sensory profile. Moreover, with age, the strategy that was very useful for this particular child may not work anymore and should be replaced by another one to reflect the changes in the person's abilities to function. (Some professionals insist that there is no research evidence that 'sensory treatments' work with autistic individuals as no research study has shown that any particular treatment is beneficial for all children with autism. There is no surprise here due to a huge variability of sensory problems in autism.

 ## Pause for Thought – A Painful Truth

As he grew, I began to notice more and more Alyosha's very acute aversion to some things we would not think twice about. Seemingly mundane tasks such as getting dressed or getting his nails cut were surprisingly difficult.

When it came to having his nails cut, his distress was so severe that I had to start being creative to get it done. So, when he was asleep, I would have to creep quietly into his room to accomplish the task. It probably wasn't the best option, but the only other one was for a friend (or two) to hold him down whilst I cut his nails, listening to his screaming protests.

Of course, anybody could see this was a highly uncomfortable situation for my son – but nobody could tell me why he was so distressed. Was it a fear of the scissors or was it the sensation of the scissors against the nail?

I needed to find out, because not understanding your own son and what puts him in such stress is hugely upsetting. Once I delved deeper, I found that for the majority of autistic people, the sense of touch is highly acute. Not even that but the duration of this sensation can last for hours, days and even weeks.

These sensations can be explained thanks to modern neurological research where comparative studies have been done with autistic and non-autistic individuals. Research found that in autistic individuals, transmitted sensory information was not contained in small units in the brain (called 'minicolumns'*), but instead 'overflowed' to nearby units, creating an amplifier effect[6].

Professor Manuel Casanova compares these inhibitory fibres with a shower curtain. When working properly and fully protecting the bathtub, the shower curtain prevents water from spilling to the floor. In autism, 'water is all over the bathroom'.

Sensory stimuli can be experienced very differently by autistic individuals. Just because we may not feel something, it does not mean that they don't. It's something that is so simple to understand, yet not knowing anything about it makes you feel like you know nothing and you are unable to help your own child.

Alyosha hates 'nail-cutting' as the process of 'cutting' doesn't stop when I finish clipping his nails and put the scissors away. The boy keeps feeling the sensation for at least three to four days. He tries to describe how it feels, but because of his differences and difficulties in using language, the best he comes up with is, 'My nails are sticky.' He feels better on the fifth or sixth day after the 'traumatic event', but the comfortable existence lasts only a few more days until it's time to have his nails clipped again.

Many parents of autistic children shared similar experiences with me. A common one is getting the child changed into different clothes. It is well known that autistic children insist on sameness and many prefer to wear the same clothes day in, day out. Whilst others can forget the sensation of clothes on their skin after just a few seconds (called 'habituation'*), many autistic individuals do not. The habituation process does not work properly for them and that is why the sensation of something on their skin may last for hours or even days.

Normally, when the senses are exposed to a continuing stimulus, whether smell, taste or touch, habituation soon occurs and the brain 'forgets' about the sensation. Just imagine what it must be like to always feel clothes on your body, and when after a few days, you gradually lose this sensation and become comfortable, it's time to change your clothes again. And it's not only daily clothes that can cause problems. For some, it can take weeks to get used to exposing the skin and to wearing shorts/skirts and short-sleeved tops in summer. But by the time they feel comfortable in summer outfits, it's autumn and time to start wearing trousers and long-sleeved jumpers again!

My son has gradually got used to these experiences, from getting dressed in new clothes to having his hair or nails cut, and he now deals with it much better than before. The sensations are still the same for him but his way of dealing with it has significantly improved. Instead of having three people holding him down, and me trying to distract him when a hairdresser started to cut his hair, we now take him to a local hairdresser who knows him well and Alyosha is able to sit through it calmly and happily. (And for the first time - at the age of 28 - he even asked the hairdresser to make "this" shorter (pointing at the unruly curl on his forehead).

Not only have I learnt more about his experiences, but I have also learnt how to be able to communicate with him about them. Now, when he asks me: "Mum, will my nails be sticky when you cut them?" I reply: "Yes, your nails will be sticky, but this feeling will pass." So, with his language and my understanding, the process is now a lot more bearable for both of us. Looking back, I've realised that over the years it wasn't only me learning how to cope with all of this. He was, too.

3

WHY IS AUTISM A PUZZLE?

T he metaphor of a jigsaw puzzle (or, rather a selection of jigsaw pieces) has been chosen by many parent and professional organisations to reflect one of the most visible traits in autism. Autistic children notice the tiniest details of places, objects, people – and often react to one 'piece' of the person or place instead of the whole situation.

I experienced this in the first few months of my son's life when I was feeding him. I used to wear the same red dressing gown and it was always the same ritual that allowed me to bond with my baby quietly and in peace. That was, until one day when I changed my outfit. That day I wore blue.

What followed was one of the worst meltdowns I had ever seen with him. He was screaming and protesting so loudly that it wasn't just the neighbours in our block of flats I was worried about, but the ones on the other side of the street, too. Luckily, instead of alerting the police, one of them decided to check on us and to see for herself what was going on. She knocked at the door and asked me if everything was alright. She sure knew it wasn't, but reassured that I wasn't torturing my baby, she offered to help by taking Alyosha from me. Immediately, he stopped crying. Deafened by sudden silence, I regained the ability to think, looked at the puzzled neighbour and literally *saw* the answer to the riddle: she was wearing a *red* dress!

My son did not see me as a whole, he associated me with the colour red. That day he was unable to recognise me because I was not wearing the same colour gown. The "bit" of me which he usually focused on completely changed. This made me an imposter in his eyes. No wonder he was scared to death and the only thing in his disposal was his voice to show it.

That was my first indication that Alyosha saw 'in bits' (fragmented vision) and could consciously process only certain fragments of his surroundings. When these were subject to change, he would feel frightened and disoriented. Troublesome behaviour would soon follow.

When he got older, his language made me realise his perception was indeed very different. So, I wasn't surprised when I heard him reporting, for example, that 'the cat's head has turned round.'

With this type of processing, Alyosha had great difficulty in dealing with people, as they seemed to comprise of both unconnected pieces and unpredictable movements of these 'bits of people'. His strategy to cope with the problem was to avoid people and never look at them. It wasn't that he couldn't *see* an entire person, rather he was unable to *process* the meaning of an entire person – and would do this bit by bit instead. As a result, the mental image of a 'collection of bits' was meaningless and often frightening.

The worst were hands and arms. People tend to move or wave their hands while talking or pointing (especially teachers at school). Their hands seemed to be unconnected. He hated it when somebody pointed at things to attract his attention, as a disconnected hand suddenly appearing from nowhere (and belonging to nobody) in front of him could scare him and trigger "aggression" – a protective reaction (from his point of view).

Alyosha instinctively tried to calm himself during these times of anxiety by flapping his hands in front of his eyes. This helped him to ignore many 'offending' and confusing stimuli around him. His other strategy in times of sensory overload was to focus on one object in the environment – the item he would choose as a recognizable 'bit' of this particular place, event or situation. If this item had been unintentionally removed, it could lead to a panic attack as he couldn't identify the place or situation and everything became unpredictable (and, therefore, dangerous).

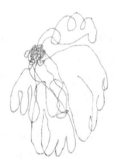

Alyosha's drawing of hands shows this.

Fragmentation was not limited to vision. He would describe how his body would break into "many little pieces" at night. Alyosha was also sure that he had two foreheads and for many years asked me to kiss both good night ('this one and that one').

* * * * *

 Notes in the Margin – Perception 'in bits'

Perception 'in bits' means that autistic children define people, places and objects by these bits. They can suddenly find once familiar things to be strikingly unfamiliar if slight components are changed, such as when the furniture has been moved or someone doesn't wear the same dress as usual. As they process what they perceive piece by piece and not as a whole, they recognise things and people by the 'sensory pieces' they store as their definitions. For instance, they may recognise people and objects by smell, sound, intonation, the way they move and so on.

So, many 'images' (bits and pieces) have to be re-assembled to get a whole picture of the environment. These 'bits' jump out at them. A colour or shape can catch their attention, then some other detail will float into their focus, thus, detail by detail they have to sort them out, mentally deciding why all these fragments go so close together (though what is 'in front of', what is 'behind', 'on', 'next to' is not clear at this stage), eventually seeing / interpreting one picture.

The fragmented perception can affect all the senses: some children (with 'fragmented vision') may recognise their mother by smell, or by her voice; or they may be attracted by an earring or glasses on somebody's face without paying attention to the person (or sometimes even not realising that there is a person in front of them). The result is that autistic children often react upon parts of objects or people as being complete entities: a hand (unattached to anyone), a foot and so on.

It is difficult to identify the 'sensory concepts' the child uses to function in the environment. However, some parents intuitively know what might upset their child.

 ## There's always a BUT – Delayed Processing

As a consequence of a fragmented perception, autistic children may experience a delayed response to sensory stimuli; for example, you say something to your child, and there is no response as if the child didn't hear you. However, actually the child has started to process your question/instruction in order to respond with meaning, but he may need some time to process the question and prepare his response.

Working with my students I noticed that the immediate response to my questions/instructions was often automatic (triggered by memories) and not necessarily what they meant. It looked like they were not listening. If I tried to help them by repeating the question or rephrasing it, I confused them completely. Repeating the same question interrupts the processing of the 'first question', and the child must start all over again because 'the same (but yet unprocessed) question' is a new one for them. In other words, an interruption effectively wipes away any intermediate result, confronting the autistic child literally *for the first time* with the same object/event/situation.

So I learned very early in my teaching career not to rush them and give them time to respond. If there was no immediate response it didn't mean that the question went unnoticed – it had been sensed and recorded without interpretation until the second (internalised) hearing (i.e., processing of the received message).

They may be able to repeat back what has been said without comprehension that will come later. In less extreme cases, to process something takes seconds or minutes. But sometimes it takes days, weeks, or months. In the most extreme cases, it can take years to process what has been said. The words, phrases, sentences, and sometimes the whole situations are stored and they can be triggered at any time. You must be a detective to connect the child's 'announcement' with the question he/she was asked a week before. For example, Alyosha sometimes gave responses a few days later. (For an outsider, his responses, unconnected to the present situation, seemed weird.)

A child can be delayed on every sensory channel.
There are several consequences of delayed processing:
· They are often unable to start the action immediately as they need time to interpret and comprehend the situation.

· When they finally reach comprehension, the situation has changed. It means that they experience meaning out of the context it should have been experienced in. That is why, new experiences, no matter how similar to previous ones, are perceived as new, unfamiliar and unpredictable, and responses to them are poor regardless of the number of times the child has experienced the same thing.

· The amount of time needed to process any experience often remains slow (or delayed) regardless of having had similar experiences in the past; things do not get easier with time or learning[7].

Do's and Dont's

As some children with autism perceive everything in pieces, they need time to adjust to different surroundings. As the number of objects seen by them is greater (because they sometimes perceive different images for the same object from different angles), they do not feel safe in the constantly changing environment.

- Structure* makes the environment predictable and easier to control.
- Routine and rituals help to facilitate understanding of what is going on and what is going to happen.
- Introduce any change very slowly and always explain beforehand what is happening differently and why.
- Give them time to take in your question/instruction and to work out their response. Do not interrupt. Be aware that autistic individuals often require more time than others to shift their attention between stimuli of

different modalities and they find it extremely difficult to follow rapidly changing social interactions.

 ## Pause for Thought – Learning About Theories – Be Critical

There are many different theories attempting to explain autism. All of them contain some very interesting (and useful) ideas but none explain the autistic condition in its entirety. Many authors employ metaphorical descriptions to make their theory easier to understand. However, metaphorical interpretation can also be misleading.

Learning about theories of autism (even if they are not correct) has helped me find solutions to many riddles my son presents me with. However, understanding that autistic children often perceive the world around them in fragments didn't answer a very important question – why don't they 'see the whole picture'?

One of the theories claiming to explain the phenomenon is weak central coherence (WCC) theory: people with autism lack the 'built-in form of coherence' and, as a result, they see the world as fragmented. This theory was suggested by Uta Frith (who explained it in her book with a very ambitious title – *Autism: Explaining the Enigma*). The metaphorical frame sounds nice. However, certain questions should have been asked but weren't: What exactly is 'built-in form of coherence'? Where (in the brain?) is it located/represented? How does (or doesn't) it work?, and many others. If 'central coherence' exists (or is lacking in autism) it must have some real qualities and characteristics. So what does it look like? I've asked my friends and challenged them to visualise and describe (or draw) it. The results were interesting: Most showed it with their hands, commenting 'Well, it's like pulling everything together'/ 'It's something in the brain'/ 'It's like this' (moving hands in circles).

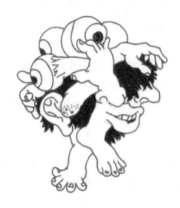

Ian Wilson: 'Built-in form of coherence'

In fact, autistic children do see the full picture alright – the trouble is that they perceive too much! What their brain cannot do is to simplify for the sake of coherence. In non-autistic people, the brain omits large chunks of information and generalises in order to make sense of experiences. In autistic people who experience sensory overload, no such filter is available.

Later, my own research showed that in contrast to the WCC hypothesis, autistic children possess a very strong drive for coherence – caused by the lack of sensory filters – that is reflected in gestalt perception*.

It sounds illogical but it does make sense. As too much information needs to be processed simultaneously (and no brain is capable of that), they often select for attention minor aspects of objects in the environment instead of the whole scene or person (that's where the WCC explanation fits in nicely). For example, where we may see a room, an autistic child sees a door handle, a leg of the table, a coin on the floor or a piece of fluff on the carpet.

4

EVERY TINY THING IS IMPORTANT

It's a common mistake - to oversimplify sensory problems in autism, reducing them to hyper- and hyposensitivities. It is not enough to identify the hypersensitive sensory channel(s) and adjust the environment to make it easier for the child to tolerate.

It turns out to be much more complicated, as hypersensitivities in autism are merely the consequences of other sensory perceptual differences, which may include the inability to filter sensory information, monoprocessing, fragmentation, delayed processing, peripheral perception and others.

One of my first pupils, Pavlik (7 years old), constantly informed me about what was going on in other rooms in the building or outside. It went like this:

Me: "There are seven days in a week: Sunday..."
Pavlik (interrupting me): "Somebody's opened the window on the ground floor. Are they hot?"
- Monday, Tuesday...
- They are moving the chairs around the room downstairs. Why?

His brain seemed to try to process all the stimuli around him: to my 'Wednesday' I got 'Who is coughing outside? And to 'Friday' it was 'Someone's walking in the corridor'... His inability to screen out all the irrelevant noises and sounds (even those no one else could hear) meant that he couldn't make sense of what was going on in our classroom. His ears picked up all the sounds with equal intensity. The boy got easily frustrated when trying to do something in a noisy, crowded room. He didn't seem to understand my questions or instructions if someone else was talking in the same room.

My students had to 'put everything right' in the classroom (the way it was the day before) and only then we could start our lessons. For them, each and every situation was unique. They could perform in the exactly same environment with the exactly same prompts but fail to apply the skill if anything in the environment, routine or prompt was (even slightly) changed. For instance, Helen could recite her multiplication tables if I put my hand on her shoulder and was unable to give any answer if no prompt was provided. And she couldn't do it with her mum at home.

My pupils made their own connections (causes and effects) and considered them as universal laws. During break times, the door to the kitchen was usually shut, and if Alyosha happened to find it open after lunch, he didn't know what to do in this situation. If the door is open, does it mean another lunch?

Another confusing (and frightening) thing for them was when something (or somebody) emerged in the situation that didn't belong to it; for example, if they encountered their doctor in the supermarket. (Some wouldn't even recognise her.) At our 'social interaction classes' I could teach them what to do and what to say in different social situations, but if someone else was present and wanted to join in, they were lost, upset or anxious. The 'wrong voice', the 'wrong words' confused and baffled them.

Each of my students had their own ritualistic behaviours. These routines brought reassurance and order in their daily life, which was otherwise unpredictable and threatening. Some rituals were long and complicated, for instance, every morning Sasha entered the classroom and touched each chair, then looked out of the window and tapped the window-sill several times before he settled at his desk. I had to explain to 'outsiders' that for the boy it was *one* act of meaningful experience, and if any part of it was missing (for example, Sasha was prevented from tapping the window-sill or touching one of the chairs) the whole experience became incomplete, unfamiliar, and frightening, – and he would need to start again from the very beginning.

When my son was younger, it was impossible to return from a walk with him without following exactly the same path and stopping at the same places we'd done before. To avoid any major accident, I learnt to cover the same ground when we went out. If we met someone, while we were walking in the park or on the street, and I stopped to talk to the person, Alyosha used to throw himself down on the ground (or a puddle if it was raining) screaming his head off. If it happened in a 'safe place' (not on the road, e.g.), the best strategy was to wait for him to calm down – standing next to him – protecting him from people passing by and the people from his "kicks" and himself from injuries. Nothing else would work – he wasn't in control.

More problems emerged when we went, for example, shopping by car. I don't know about other countries but in the UK, roadworks seem to be a British institution – wherever and whenever we drive, there are road-workers digging (or filling in) the holes. For Alyosha and others like him, it's very confusing (why do we turn right when we are supposed to go straight ahead?) and frightening (are we going where Mother said we'd go?).

In addition, small parts of a routine may carry huge significance. Whereas for most, leaving the day centre building at a certain time meant that the day was over, for Alyosha it was only complete when he had shut the centre's door. This routine was interrupted recently and a very distressing meltdown, lasting some hours, followed. After we had recovered and I was able to unravel the day, I understood what had caused it.

There is a (seeming) paradox in autism: many children cope with big changes much better than with tiny ones. The matter is, a new place and situation is, in fact, a new gestalt, and they will remember it. (For example, our first holiday in Greece was very successful, so we decided to go there again in two years' time. The first thing Alyosha did when we entered the (same) hotel was dropping on all fours and crawling under the armchair in the lobby – where he lost his toy two years before.) However, any tiny change in his bedroom (without him being present) brings anxiety – something is wrong, the bedroom doesn't feel the same.

* * * * *

Notes in the Margin – Problems with screening out irrelevant stimuli

The inability to filter foreground and background information (and perception of the whole scene as a single entity with all the details perceived – not processed! – simultaneously) can be called gestalt perception. Autistic children may experience it in any sensory modality. A child with auditory gestalt perception has a great difficulty to focus on one auditory stimulus, for example, someone's voice, as it is heard with all the other environmental noises: fans working, doors opening, somebody coughing, cars passing, etc. If they try to screen out the background noise, they also screen out the voice they are trying to attend to. Individuals with visual gestalt perception experience all visual stimuli (details) around them simultaneously.

Without efficient filtering and selectivity of attention, the child cannot make sense of the environment. Autistic children are often unable to divide their attention between the object they want and the person whom they are supposed to ask for it because for many of them, shifting attention from one stimulus to the other is a relatively slow process. Another common attentional problem in autism is the failure of autistic children to establish and maintain joint attention, i.e., the ability to attend to the same stimuli as another person. That leads to failure to share experiences. This, in turn, results in the difficulty to comprehend the meaning of the interaction and hinder social and cultural development.

Gestalt perception accounts for their dislike of changes and insistence on 'sameness'. If the slightest detail is changed (for instance, a picture on the wall is not straight, or a piece of furniture has been moved a few inches to the side), the whole scene is different, i.e., unfamiliar. The same is true about routines: if something goes differently, they do not know what to do. Gestalt of the situation is different. All this results in fear, stress and frustration. To feel safe in their environment, these children need sameness and predictability.

 There's always a BUT – Difficulties caused by the inability to filter sensory information

Autistic children are easily overloaded in situations which, for us, are 'normal' – for example, in supermarkets, crowded places, or even 'normal classrooms'. The difficulty to filter the incoming stimulation (and being overwhelmed by it) makes it hard for the children to integrate into their peer group and restricts their ability to understand what is going on around them.

Being aware of gestalt perception can help us understand and address the difficulties caused by it:

- *Insistence on sameness, resistance to change*: any tiny change results in a completely 'new picture' (gestalt), making learned skills inapplicable.

- *Difficulty generalising knowledge*: it's impossible to single out a few connections (that are supposed to be relevant/significant to each situation) if the 'picture'/template doesn't correspond to the one they know.

- *Rejecting new things and activities; preference for what they have experienced and known*: any new activity or situation demands new solutions that are not known yet.

- *Imposition of routines and rituals*: even if they don't know what to do, the rituals and routines reassure them that everything goes the way it should.

- *Difficulty in making choices*: there is so much to consider, so it's easier to choose something they know, or to follow somebody else's choice.

- *Lack of compliance*: if the child is unprepared and doesn't know what's going on or the situation/activity is new, the best strategy is to refuse to participate in /do it.

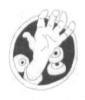

Do's and Dont's

The ways in which we can help them sort out sensory information are:

- find out which sensory modality does not filter information and make the environment 'visually/auditorily, etc. simple';

- always monitor the number of simultaneous stimuli and reduce all irrelevant stimuli. If there are several conversations in the same room, plus air conditioning switched on, plus people moving around, plus the fridge switched on in the kitchen... the person with sensory hypersensitivities is likely to be overwhelmed. The same goes for bright light, colours, tactile stimuli, smells, etc.

- create structure (of time, place and activity) and routine to make the environment predictable and easier to control; it will make understanding of everyday activities easier and provide feeling of safety and trust;

- give explicit instructions, highlighting each step in the completion of the task, by providing a sample of the final product – for the child to see what is expected from him/her;

- teach the same skills in different situations, with different people, in different places; provide as many opportunities as possible – for them to learn to generalise their knowledge and to use their skills in different situations, in different places, with different people;

- show the connections with previous activities and skills explicitly;

- always communicate to the child beforehand, in a way he/she can understand (for instance, using verbal, visual, tactile, etc. means) what and why will be changed. For example, tell the child what will happen the day before, then in the morning, half or a quarter of an hour before this new event/activity. Some children will need less time to 'get used to' the idea of what will happen, others – more.

Changes in the child's environment (e.g., in the bedroom or the classroom) should be with the child's active participation.

Good news is: though it won't happen overnight, with experience (and support) they do learn to be flexible. (But do remember you have to become flexible yourself – be prepared to change your schedule/methods/attitude when the child needs it.)

Pause for Thought – Are all Autistics Savants?

There is another side of the gestalt phenomenon that can be seen as a strength. We can find the best illustration of it in the works of autistic savants – those who can produce beautiful drawings or repeat any musical piece after they've heard it only once. For example, Peter Myers, an outstanding artist with Asperger syndrome produces drawings showing a great attention to details:

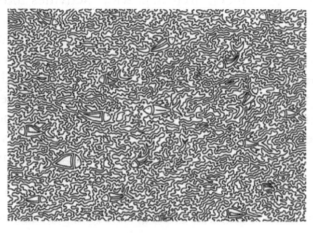

Peter Myers 'Fish in water'

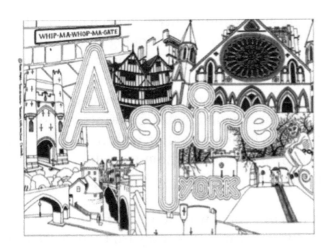

Peter Myers 'York, England'

Savant syndrome

Savant syndrome is thought to be a rare but extraordinary condition in which individuals with serious mental disabilities have some 'islands of genius'. Areas of skills traditionally attributed to savants are musical and artistic ability, an exceptional memory for spelling, mathematical abilities, calendar calculation, geographical abilities (reading maps, remembering directions, locating places), mechanical abilities (taking apart and putting together complex mechanical and electric equipment), a remarkable ability to balance objects with great accuracy) and outstanding knowledge in a specific field (such as, for example, history, statistics).

Individuals with savant skills are often able to perform tasks better than 'normal' people.

One can say it's impossible to compare autistic savants or high-functioning autistic individuals with so-called low-functioning autistic children. However, the principle of perception is the same – the whole scene (with all the tiny details) is perceived as one entity.

47

There are just two differences between people like Peter Myers and so-called low-functioning autistic individuals. First, people, like Peter, are not easily overwhelmed by unfiltered stimuli but rather take them all in and store them in their memory, while others can't cope with the sensory bombardment. Second, autistic savants can reproduce the images (whether visual or auditory) and these are spectacular, while those whom we call low-functioning can't do that.

Only 10% of people with autism are said to have savant skills. However, if we move away from 'spectacular skills' (like the ability to perform a musical piece after hearing it only once, or outstanding drawing abilities, or calendar calculating), we will see that due to the differences of their sensory perceptual and cognitive processes, *all* individuals with autism can do something non-autistic people cannot. Donna Williams[8] states that 'savant skills' can and do extend beyond art, music and 'calendar memories' and may include mimicry, speed-reading, automatic writing, the acquisition of foreign languages and others.

Unlike 'recognised savant skills' (that are spectacular because 'normal' people can achieve them only with a lot of practice and hard work), other skills that only autistic individuals possess are not recognised because the 'normal' population cannot even imagine that they exist. For example, 'sensing time':

My son cannot tell the time (I've spent hours teaching him how to 'read' time but didn't succeed) but he seems to 'sense' it. Thus, he left me baffled when one day, he said, "My clock is ten minutes slow". (I have to explain here that we had only one clock and it was in his room, the rest of us used wrist watches. He had (and has) no mobile phone or computer to see the 'right' time.) First, I thought he was just confused and didn't know what he was talking about, but then I went into his room, looked at his clock (and then at my watch) and found that he was absolutely right – his clock was ten minutes slow! It was time to replace the battery.

There have been other strange cases that I cannot explain. Like, for example, when Alyosha was 11, we were in the Lake District and I asked my partner what time it was, and before he could answer, our son loudly announced 'Quarter past two!' Need I say that it was quarter past two? Of course, the first explanation that sprang in my mind was 'it's just a coincidence,' but there have been so many coincidences since then that it begs a question: Are they coincidences, or is he able to sense the time?

5

—.—

RED ALERT: INCOMING SENSORY MISSILES...

At the time of my ignorance about autism, I remember how proud I was of some Alyosha's 'oddities' (rarely, if ever, observed in my friends' children of the same age). My son was very tidy: he would avoid messy things and places, never stepped on the puddle or touched anything if he wasn't familiar with the texture of it. However, when Alyosha started talking, some of his 'announcements' were also different from other children, and my pride gave way to puzzlement. For example, my boy often complained of 'moths' flying around him. Years later I realised that his vision was so hypersensitive that he could see particles in the air which became the foreground with the rest of his environment fading away. My son's vision was very acute (hyper-): he could see the smallest pieces of fluff on the carpet, disliked bright colours and was frightened by sharp flashes of light. The sensory overload caused by bright lights, fluorescent lights, some colours and patterns made his whole body react as if it was being attacked, resulting in negative biochemical changes, which often led to such physical symptoms as headaches, anxiety, panic attacks and 'aggression'. These experiences distracted his attention from whatever he was supposed to do. To lessen the stress caused by 'visual bombardment', Alyosha used his 'defensive visual behaviours': looking away, looking in short glances, looking through fingers, looking down, or shutting down his visual channel altogether.

What made things even more complicated was that his hearing was also very acute: the boy seemed to hear noises before others became aware of any sound; for example, he informed me about his dad coming home before I would spot the car turning to the porch. (Even now, as noises seem so much louder to him, Alyosha tends to move away from conversations and avoids crowded places.)

Hypersensitivities to sensory stimuli are very common in autism. During the years, I've worked with children with various hypersensitivities. Several students (including my son) in my class were hypersensitive to fluorescent light: they could see a 50-cycle flickering, making the room pulsate on and off. However, their reactions to it were different: some tried to escape – running out of the room, while Dima... fell asleep.

Inna (with *smell hypersensitivities*) ran from smells. We banned perfume on the premises but, unfortunately, it was not good enough – at lunch break the odours from some food were too strong for her. (At home she had a very special diet of 'unsmelly food'.)

If it was raining, Sasha (with *auditory hypersensitivity*) was likely to miss his classes – the sound of thunder (physically!) hurt his ears, and he refused point blank to leave his flat – sitting on his bed (sometimes, crawling under the bed) with his index fingers pushed into his ears.

However, often, *auditory hypersensitivity* isn't necessarily about loud sounds; sometimes the most disturbing sounds for an autistic individual are those that cannot be heard by non-autistic people. They might cover their ears when the noise is painful for them, though others in the same room may be unaware of any disturbing sounds at all. Sometimes *hyperauditory* children make repetitive noises to block out other disturbing sounds.

Vita was *hypertactile*: she couldn't tolerate hugs; and washing her hair was an ordeal, demanding several people to complete it. She also overreacted to heat/cold and didn't like wearing shoes.

Pete refused to wear silk shirts because he couldn't tolerate the fabric on his skin. His parents learned to accommodate this, because if they forced him to wear a silk top, the boy would strip the offending item off at the earliest opportunity – on the bus, in the town centre or at school.

Children with *proprioceptive hypersensitivity* hold their bodies in odd positions, have difficulty manipulating small objects, etc. Those with *vestibular hypersensitivity* have a low tolerance for any activity that involves movement or quick change in the position of the body; experience difficulty changing directions and walking or crawling on uneven or unstable surfaces. They are poor at sports; feel disoriented after spinning, jumping or running and often express fear and anxiety of having their feet leave the ground.

Autistic children are vulnerable to being abused.They have to live in a world which is not designedfor them. If we look at their 'bizarre' behaviours and responses through their eyes, they make sense. Our behaviours may equally seem 'bizarre' to autistic children. For instance, how could one enjoy fireworks if your eyes are hit with 'bunches of bright arrows' and the sound in your ears 'tears them raw'? We often do not understand the 'autistic perspective', the problems they experience. And sometimes our 'treatment' does more harm than good. For example:

A family were struggling to find the solution to a challenging behaviour of an eight-year-old autistic boy. He removed his clothes at any opportunity no matter where he was. The mother asked for advice from a 'specialist'. And the advice was to encourage the boy to keep his clothes on and reward him (with a chocolate biscuit) when he complied. If we look at this situation from the 'autistic perspective', tactile hypersensitivity is obvious. The boy himself was aware of which fabric would hurt him and tried to protect himself. His clues were not recognized by the people involved. Wasn't it more logical (and beneficial to the child) to identify the fabrics the boy couldn't tolerate and provide him with the clothes he felt comfortable with, while desensitizing his tactile system?

* * * * *

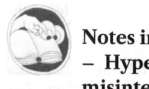

Notes in the Margin
– Hypersensitivities
misinterpreted as ESP

Sometimes sensory hypersensitivities are misinterpreted as extrasensory perception (ESP) as 'normal' people not only fail to see, hear, smell or feel what some autistic individuals can, but also find it hard to imagine that these experiences are possible because 'normal' people are blind, deaf and dumb to the stimuli which are everyday experiences for some autistic individuals. However, there is *nothing* extrasensory about their ability to hypersense as some autistic people's senses are so acute that they may see, hear, feel or smell the stimuli that are undetectable by the majority. Their senses are finely tuned to the environment. For example, some react to tiny changes in weather patterns and atmosphere pressure; others can *see* energy and its movement around them. Many are sensitive to vibration or sensitive to small differences in colour, have enhanced auditory discrimination as if their brains are tuned to higher frequencies. Some autistic children can hear some frequencies that only animals can hear. (By the way, we don't assume that animals have ESP, do we?)

Why don't we appreciate their ability (caused by their heightened senses) to perceive (and experience) colour, sound, texture, smell and taste to a higher degree than people around them? The answer is simple – how can we appreciate something if we have never experienced it? – It's easier to assume it doesn't exist.

The ability to hypersense can lead to a hypnotic level of hypersensation: a typical picture of an autistic child is when he/she is staring transfixed at something: watching the reflection of light, colour or visual patterns, or absorbed with vibration of sounds, or constantly touching objects of certain texture. In this sense, autistic perception can be seen as superior to that of the majority whose senses function 'normally'. However, the longer someone stays in this hypnotic state, the more addictive it becomes, and the person may miss out on developing social skills and experiencing the life of the majority.

 ## There's always a BUT – Any sudden unpredictable stimuli can be painful

Have you ever thought that it's possible to hurt (physically!) someone by just switching on fluorescent light in the room? Or hit someone with certain sounds? And even if the child asks us not to hurt him, do we listen?

For instance, at one of the autistic provisions, a teaching support assistant is happily whistling and singing; Joe, an 11-year-old autistic boy, is rocking back and forth. He covers his ears with his hands, but it does not seem to work and he pushes his index fingers inside his ears. No effect. Then he pleads with his 'helper': 'Laura, stop singing, please. Stop it!' The reaction of the support worker? 'Why should I? Don't be stupid, Joe.' If we look at the same situation from Joe's perspective, we could see it as a sensory assault of the child. For this boy, the 'singing' (whether it was the pitch of the voice or the sounds of whistling he could not tolerate) physically hurt his ears, as if the helper was hitting him with a heavy object. So why should she stop?

Not only certain stimuli but also *any sudden unpredictable* stimuli can be painful. Some children will break telephones because, if they are not prepared to the sudden sound, telephone ringing may startle them.

When he was younger, Alyosha would 'attack' babies because he couldn't tolerate the pitch of the voices. And what's more he would try to hit a baby, even if the baby was asleep. It seems illogical, but, in fact, it's a very logical and (though it sounds horrible) rational behaviour: babies are unpredictable, and if they suddenly start crying the boy would jump out of his skin as the pain would be unbearable, so (from his point of view) it was logical to initiate the crying when he was prepared for it.

Do's and Dont's

If the child is hypersensitive, even a 'visually/auditorily' quiet environment may cause overstimulation and challenges for the child. Autistic children must be protected from painful stimuli.

· Remember, what we think is enjoyable (for example, fireworks) may be fearful or overwhelming to an autistic child. We should always bear in mind that if we cannot hear/see/smell/feel some stimuli, it does not mean that the child 'is being stupid' if distressed by 'nothing'.

· Identify which sensory stimuli may interfere with the individual's capability to cope and either reduce them or eliminate them, or, if impossible, provide the 'sensory aids' (for example, tinted glasses, earplugs) to protect them from painful sensory bombardment.

· Desensitise the child to tolerate the stimuli via a sensory diet: We can adjust the environment at home and at school to protect the child from painful stimuli but to keep him/her in these safe places 24/7 is not an option because we want to give our children the best possible chance to fully participate in all activities and to be a part of the community

Desensitisation is supposed to increase sensory tolerance very gradually through sensory activities (so called *sensory diets*) – prescribed by the occupational therapist. These activities are aimed to raise the child's threshold for arousal. They are never forced but introduced gently in the form of games and pleasurable exercises. The therapist typically analyses the child's processing of sensations of different sensory modalities in relation to the child's ability to learn and move, and then incorporates meaningful activities that provide specific sensory stimuli to elicit an adaptive response, thereby assisting the child in overall motor and conceptual learning.

An occupational therapist teaches the parents to use these techniques with a child at home for three to five minutes, six to eight times a day. As the child starts responding, for example, to touch more normally, the time of the sessions is reduced. The therapist should monitor the child's responsiveness to the strategies and, if any adverse reactions occur, the therapist discontinues the activity and modifies the treatment accordingly.

In case of *visual hypersensitivity*, there are several methods to help: for instance, fluorescent lights might be replaced by ordinary bulbs. Tinted glasses can improve visual perception of the environment. The optimal colour is very individual and depends on each person's unique visual-perceptual sensitivities. It seems that the coloured lenses filter out those frequencies of the light spectrum to which the person may be uniquely sensitive: the use of colour appears to change the rate at which visual information is processed by the brain, thus reducing overload and hypersensitivity.

Other positive changes are perception with depth instead of seeing a two-dimensional world, no fragmentation of visual information, improvement in eye contact, the ability to use several channels at the same time (for example, to see *and* hear); reduced sensitivity to auditory stimuli, increased ability to understand language, and better fine and gross motor coordination. As vision becomes a reliable sense, there is no need to use other senses to compensate, so there is better processing of sound, touch and body awareness.

Strategies to accommodate for *auditory sensitivities* are: headphones to listen to calming music; earplugs to reduce extraneous auditory stimuli. However, these devices should be used only short-term (for noisy places) because habitual use of them may bring considerable problems with the opposite effect – increased hypersensitivity.

There are other approaches to address hyperauditory problems, for instance, the Tomatis Method and Berard's Auditory Integration Training (AIT)*; both methods have been reported beneficial, but there is still some controversy in the reports: some say that the benefits were short-lived, others could see improvements not only in reducing auditory sensitivities but also improvements in other sensory systems. Though training a person's hearing to not perceive disturbing frequencies may bring reduction of stress in the short term for some people, it will not necessarily improve the efficiency of information processing and sensory overload. This could be addressed equally well by using ear plugs in noisy places and reducing the number of simultaneous stimuli.

Another technique to address specific sound sensitivities is exposure therapy*. Though designed to treat phobias[9], it has been used with autistic children. It aims to desensitise the child by exposing him to disturbing sounds – first at a distance but gradually closer and closer to the child. A version of this technique is using recorded offending sounds and letting the child to be in control: initiating the sound and gradually increasing its volume and stopping the exercise altogether at any time.

Tactile hypersensitivities should be addressed by choosing the clothes and fabrics the child can tolerate. As people with hypertactility are frightened by light touch, especially if it is unpredictable, always approach the child from the front to prepare him/her visually for possible touch.

Different techniques are used to address hypersensitivity to touch, for example, the Deep Pressure Proprioceptive Touch Technique which involves the use of a small brush and a massage protocol. With a special brush, the therapist makes firm, brisk movements over the body, especially the arms, hands, legs and feet. The brushing is followed by a technique of deep joint compression. As the child receives deep touch pressure, the tactile receptors that are hypersensitive to light touch are depressed. Touch sensitivity can also be reduced by massaging the body. Eventually, the child's tolerance to tactile stimulation increases.

Many autistic children and adults like deep pressure. It is easy to apply comforting dark pressure over large areas of the body to little children by placing them under large pillows or rolling them up in heavy gym mats. There are specially devised vests for individuals of different ages to apply pressure to the body, and 'heavy blankets' – to help them sleep.

Other approaches to address tactile and proprioceptive problems are holding therapy* and a hug/squeeze machine* (which was designed by Temple Grandin). One of the assumptions in holding therapy is that when held safely in his mother's arms, the autistic child learns to overcome the fear of direct eye contact and close attachment[10].

However, holding therapy assumes that all sensory and perceptual systems are intact and integrated and that information processing for the person is basically 'normal', except that issues like 'love' and who is in control have not yet been established for that person[11]. The same (or even better) beneficial effect could be achieved by less stressful methods.

Temple Grandin who is very hypersensitive to touch has discovered that deep pressure can help her reduce this hypersensitivity and the anxiety it causes. She could not get the 'right' amount of pressure from people because they were uncontrollable and either gave her too much or too little deep pressure. Grandin then designed and built her own device to administer pressure and control the amount and duration of it to achieve this calming effect. Gradually she was able to tolerate the machine holding her and her hypersensitivity to touch was slowly reduced, and another positive effect was to become more social. Studies of the effectiveness of the 'hug machine' have produced some positive results. The researchers found a reduction of tension and anxiety resulted from the 'hug sessions'; the number of stereotypies decreased and more relaxed behaviour followed afterwards. The best candidates to use the machine are those with tactile hypersensitivity, hyposensitivity (seeking for deep pressure experiences) and those who cannot regulate their arousal state. Some people need time to desensitise themselves while inside the machine (letting the sides to touch them). When the nervous system becomes desensitised through gradual and slow stimulation, experience of touch becomes pleasurable.

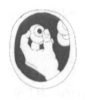 ## Pause for Thought – Why Does a 'Sensory Treatment' Work for Some Children and Doesn't Work or Even Harms Others?

We know that many people with autism do suffer from auditory problems (especially hypersensitivity to certain sounds). The AIT is aimed to reduce this hypersensitivity by retraining the ear to tolerate certain frequencies and pitches. However, we always should address the causes of auditory hypersensitivity and not the symptoms *per se*. Very often hypersensitivity is caused not by certain frequencies or certain sounds but by the number of auditory stimuli, the rate of the auditory processing the person can cope with and even other 'non-auditory' stimuli (lights, movements, etc.) that can contribute to sensory overload and result in auditory hypersensitivity. Training the ear to tolerate certain frequencies may bring some improvement in the short-term but as it doesn't address the improvement of sensory processing of other channels that may be the main source of the child's overload, it's short lived. The AIT administered to the person whose main difficulties are rooted in auditory problems (i.e., they are the causes and not just the symptoms) may produce 'miraculous' results. When the primary problem is addressed and eliminated (or lessened) we can see immediate improvements in other systems as well, as they do not need to compensate for impaired auditory channel anymore and may do their own job.

For example, Georgiana spent the first 11 years of her life in special institutions. Her mother, Annabel Stehli[12] describes Georgie's hypersensitivities to sights and sounds in her book *The Sound of a Miracle*: Georgie's vision was hypersensitive and everything she saw was magnified; for instance, every strand of hair looked like spaghetti. Her auditory hypersensitivities brought a lot of pain: the girl heard snowflakes falling, and every drop of rain sounded like a shot from the gun. Much became clear in her "abnormal" behaviour: when it rained, Georgie screamed in pain and banged her head against the wall. After the AIT, her hypersensitivity to sound diminished and this enabled her to cope with her other perceptual problems.

However, such 'miraculous success' has been achieved by a few, while for others the treatment hasn't brought any positive results because their auditory problems might have been caused by problems in other senses, sensory overload, or other difficulties that lead to hypersensitivity.

When Alyosha was eight, we had a chance to meet Donna Williams. Sitting on the carpet in the middle of the room, Donna and I were talking, while my son was running in circles flipping his toy in front of his eyes and producing his usual vocalisations, oblivious to what was going on around him. I was sharing my concerns related to his (very) painful hearing. Suddenly Donna said, 'You know, I think he sees the world the way I did, before I started wearing Irlen glasses. Without these glasses, everything around me was fragmented. I might look at somebody and see... his nose, then his eye, then his ear... All these bits and pieces of visual information should have been pasted together in my head to produce the whole picture. The glasses help enormously. The coloured lenses 'paste' the pieces of objects and people together, freeing me from this job and giving me more opportunities to use other senses efficiently. Why don't you take your son to one of the Irlen centres? I think the tinted glasses will be very beneficial for him.'

- But I thought it's his hearing...
- No, his auditory hypersensitivity results from his visual overload. I know, I was like this.

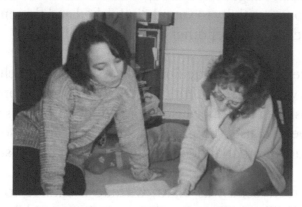

Meeting with Donna Williams, 29 February 1996

Donna interpreted my son's behaviours from his perspective and described the internal mechanisms he used to understand the world around him. It was as if I had been blind and deaf up to that moment. The newly gained eye-sight and hearing let me see (and hear) how amazing and fascinating the sensory world of autism was.

Since Alyosha started wearing his tinted lenses (at the age of nine), his light sensitivity considerably decreased, his eye contact improved from none to several seconds, and his 'visual behaviour' (using his eyes to look instead of relying on his hearing and sense of smell to 'see') significantly improved. The decrease of visual distortions and light sensitivity led to the reduction of auditory hypersensitivities, an increase of attention span, reading abilities, and the improvement of motor coordination, and of course – fewer 'challenging behaviours'.

When Alyosha reached puberty, however, there were times (and places), when even his lenses couldn't reduce the overload. For example, it was difficult for him to be in crowded places or in rooms with fluorescent lights. After 30-40 minutes, one could see that the boy wasn't coping. In these cases, his anger was directed at... his glasses. He hit them or threw them on the ground, complaining "The glasses are not working".

Fast forward 10 years – no more broken glasses, but still a huge reliance on them outside the house. Sometimes we call him 'our James Bond'.

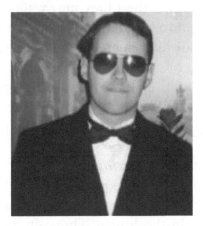

'James Bond' on a mission

6

— · —

TOO DIM, TOO QUIET, TOO 'UNFELT'...

I 've been working with children with sensory *hyposensitivities* – when their senses seem not to work properly and not enough sensory stimulation comes in, so they do not really see, hear or feel anything. To stimulate their senses, they might wave their hands around or rock back and forth or make strange noises.

Children with *hypovision* may experience trouble figuring out where objects are, as they see just outlines or colours, or shadows; then they may walk around objects running their hand around the edges so they can recognise what it is. These children are attracted to lights, they may stare at the sun or a bright light bulb. Having entered an unfamiliar room, they have to walk around it, touching everything before they settle down. Often, they sit for hours moving fingers or objects in front of the eyes.

Children with *hypohearing* may 'seek sounds' (leaning their ear against electric equipment or enjoying crowds, sirens and so on). They like kitchens and bathrooms - the noisiest places in the house. They often create sounds themselves to stimulate their hearing - banging doors, tapping things, tearing or crumpling paper in the hand, making loud rhythmic sounds.

Children with *hypotaste/hyposmell* chew and smell everything they can get (for example, grass or play dough). They mouth and lick objects, play with faeces, eat mixed food (for instance, sweet and sour) or regurgitate.

Those with *hypotactility* don't feel pain or temperature. They may not notice a wound caused by a sharp object or they are unaware of a broken bone. They are prone to self-injuries and may bite their hand or bang their head against the wall, just to feel they are alive. They like pressure, tight clothes and often crawl under heavy objects. They hug tightly and enjoy rough and tumble play. Those with hyposensitivity to temperature can put hats, boots, coats in summer, and don't wear warm clothes in winter. (I used to have to remind my son to put on a jumper, coat, scarf and gloves when it was cold outside, otherwise he just didn't bother. With time, he could decide for himself what type of clothes he needed in different seasons.)

Children with *vestibular hyposensitivity* enjoy and seek all sorts of movement and can spin or swing for a long time without being dizzy or nauseated. They often rock back and forth or move in circles while rocking their body.

Those with *proprioceptive hyposensitivity* have difficulty knowing where their bodies are in space. They bump into objects and people, stumble frequently and have a tendency to fall. Children with hypoproprioceptive system appear floppy, often lean against people, furniture and walls. They have a weak grasp and drop things.

Children with *hypointeroception* are unaware of their own body sensations; for example, they do not feel hunger (and can go without any food for hours or even days, if they are not reminded it's time to eat something); others are the opposite – they eat and eat because they don't feel when they are full. Still, others don't feel bowel movements or when their bladder is full and it's time to go to the toilet. To address Alyosha's toileting problems (after having tried all the methods available to toilet-train him), I created a 'toilet-timetable' for him: "whether you want it or not, before going to bed – go to the toilet; every morning – go to the toilet; before going out – toilet; before every meal – toilet." It worked! Remember the story at the beginning when he instructed my colleagues to go to the toilet before having refreshments? Now, you can see why.

With hyposensitive children, we're to be on a constant alert as their body doesn't let them know if they have medical problems. It's up to us to consider safety issues: for instance, pica* (when they eat inedible substances) can result in poisoning; not feeling pain (broken bones, appendicitis) can lead to very dangerous consequences.

* * * * *

Notes in the Margin – Hyposensitivities: permanent or temporary

Hyposensitivities can be permanent or temporary – caused by shutdowns (as an adaptive strategy to protect the child from sensory overload). If information overload is not diffused in time, it can result in temporal sensory agnosia*– an inability to process sensory information. In the state of sensory agnosia, interpretation of any sense can be lost; they often act as if they really were blind, deaf, numb, sometimes – 'dead'. It is a very frightening experience. Each individualdevelops his/her own strategies to cope with it.

There's always a BUT – Children with different sensitivities in one classroom

In my practice, I've often found children with hyper- or hyposensitivities sharing the same environment. The knowledge about each child's sensitivities has helped me to plan the activities and address each child's particular needs. It is often very difficult to adjust the environment to satisfy needs of several individuals as the same stimuli may cause pain in some children and bring pleasurable experiences in others.

Helen's vision was hypo-: she was attracted by any shining object, looked intensely at people (that irritated Alex, who couldn't tolerate any direct look at him) and was fascinated with mirrors. On entering the classroom, Helen walked around it touching walls and furniture before she settled down. During class, she could move her fingers in front of her face for hours. It seemed like she couldn't get enough visual stimulation and always switched on all the lights. (This was usually followed by a fight with Alex who went into meltdown every time the light was turned on.) Helen's hearing was also hypo-: she couldn't tolerate silence and constantly sought sounds, enjoyed crowded places, and if the world was too quiet for her, she would produce noise herself – banging doors, tapping things, tearing or crumpling paper in her hand, making loud rhythmic sounds.

John (hypoauditory) always joined in Helen's 'noise making'. However, his hypersensitivity to smells prevented him from coming too close to anybody, which made any activities in the kitchen nearly impossible. John couldn't tolerate how people or objects smelt, though we, around him, were not aware of any smell at all. He ran from smells and moved away from people. For him, the smell and taste of any food was too strong, and he rejected it no matter how hungry he was. He gagged easily and ate only certain food.

John sought deep pressure and liked to lie underneath sofa cushions, demanding others to sit on top of the cushions (Helen was happy to oblige). He wore really tight belts to feel the pressure.

Vita was hypersensitive to sounds, touch and smell. If she was being touched by somebody, she immediately smelt the place of touch, and more often than not, she took off her jacket or dress with this 'spoilt spot' and refused to wear it again unless it was washed. Because of her hypertactility, Vita pulled away when people tried to hug her; even the slightest touch could send her into a panic attack.

Often sensory profiles (and needs) of children are not considered if the child has the diagnosis of autism. But place children with the opposite sensitivities (i.e., very different sensory needs) into one and the same classroom, and very soon their teacher will look for another place of employment – it's just impossible to accommodate the children's diverse, and often contrasting, needs.

Do's and Dont's

If a child is hyposensitive, provide extra stimulation through the channels that do not get enough sensory stimulation from the environment. Encourage physical exercises (e.g., climbing; pushing, pulling heavy objects, jumping, running, etc.). Swinging is good for providing stimulation for a deficient vestibular system. These procedures need to be done every day, but not for hours. Depending on the children's anxiety level, some will need access to deep pressure and swinging throughout a day to calm themselves down when they become overstimulated. But if hyposensitivity is temporary (caused by overload), i.e., a protective reaction of the child to the overwhelming chaotic environment, the approach should be not to stimulate the senses but rather to reduce overload and provide structure and predictability.

Other techniques are: tactile play (shaving cream and soap foam play, play dough, etc.), 'heavy work' activities (pushing and pulling a heavy box around the room, tug-of-war games, obstacle course), 'sandwiches' when a child is placed between two couch cushions and 'squished'), vestibular activities (large therapy balls for bouncing, rolling, jumping on trampoline, etc.).

 ## Pause for Thought – An Unstable Reality

If we identify the sensitivities of each and every child we live/work with (for instance, my son's vision, hearing, tactility and the vestibular system were hypersensitive, while proprioception, including interoception* were hypo) and think we can solve their problems, we'll have to think again. Although we can address hyper- and hyposensitivities by desensitising the child and/or providing the aids to help him/her cope (in the case of hypersensitivity), or more stimulation to 'open' the affected channel (in the case of hyposensitivity), it does not always lead to the solution of the problem. The matter is, the volume of their perception is not stable, it fluctuates, and the same child can respond differently (pleasure – indifference – distress) to the same stimuli or activities.

Several types of this inconsistency can be distinguished, for example, *fluctuation between hyper- and hypo-*; and *fluctuation between hyper-/hypo- and 'normal'*.

Fluctuation between hyper- and hyposensitivity is quite common. For example, a child who appears to be deaf on one occasion may react to an everyday soundon another occasionas if it is causingacute pain; visual stimuli that may appear so bright on one occasion will on another occasion appear very dim.

The fluctuation depends on many factors, such as, for example, developmental level, physical state, severity of autistic disorder and the degree of familiarity with the environment and situations. It will also vary depending on the age and circumstances of each child, for example, the fluctuation of sound can be continual, while in other senses, fluctuations depended on the environment (in crowded and noisy places they are worse).

The impact of environmental factors (both positive and negative) will vary with the age and circumstances of each child. At times, it may appear that everything is going well, at other times the child may exhibit challenging behaviours under similar environmental conditions.

Frequent physical exercises (at least once a day) are good for both hyper- and hyposensitivities.

Another phenomenon of inconsistent perception is *fluctuation between different 'wholes'* – when a tiny change makes the environment unrecognisable, confusing and dangerous, and the learned skills become inapplicable in these 'new' surroundings. For example, it's a huge problem not only for autistic children but also for adults with autism (typically those with Asperger syndrome) who are described as 'lacking sense of direction'. Often, they cannot recognise their own house if they approach it from a different direction, or are unable to find their room in the hotel each time they've spent a day out. [I've experienced this instability all my life. I can be lost (literally!) anywhere. My partner jokes: "You cross the road from our house and you're lost." But it's not a joke for me – the environment changes all the time: from a different angle/perspective, the buildings, trees, etc. are unrecognizable. In a way, I've found a strategy to cope in such situations (persuading myself that "it's an adventure") – it helps keep panic reaction (more or less) under control, but I know that in unfamiliar places (e.g., in a hotel) it takes me up to three days to find my room from the first attempt. Before that, the corridors, rooms, doors seem to move around, so if I leave my room, and want to return immediately then this 'immediately' means 40-45 minutes of wandering around (no, the room numbers do not help). For example, I could swear that the lift was across the corridor from my room but (eventually) I found it around the corner to the left.

I have my own theory about it: perhaps I process the visual information around me not 'in the right order' – I passed the lift a couple of minutes before I reached my room but got the meaning of what happened only when I started to unlock the door, so 'my lift' (a mental image of it) was near my room.

'Life-savers'

When everything around autistic children is unstable or fragmented, it's no wonder they seek structure, predictability, rituals and routines. Many autistic children

74

are strongly attached to certain objects: a toy, a spoon, a wrapper, a twig... The list is endless. They may insist on taking the object with them wherever they go; the reason being, they feel safe when they carry it – whatever is happening around them, the object is unchanging – stable and comforting.

When going out, my son insisted on carrying something in his hand – anything would do: a toy, a twig, a leaf, a pencil, etc. – as long as it could be flapped or swung. At home the boy had his favourite toy, the removal or loss of which would cause him extreme distress.

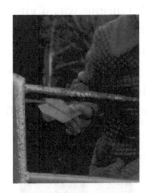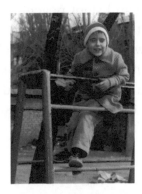

A little piece of cardboard paper provides a feeling of being protected from an unstable environment.

His need to hold a toy or any other object in his hand was obvious as if he'd been in the middle of the ocean firmly clutching at a straw to stay afloat. If nothing was available at that moment, Alyosha focused on his hands – moving them in front of his eyes. His fascination with his own hands and fingers was intriguing – he looked like a little scientist studying an extra-terrestrial object that he just happened to discover.

I always let him have a 'safety object' (a toy, a piece of string or any other object to which he seemed to have a strong attachment to) when we went to unfamiliar places or face an unfamiliar situation). One of the 'life-savers' was Gnome (which in our 'normal' world was known as 'Rudolf, the reindeer').

This little fella has saved us so many times. Gnome has never been a toy for Alyosha (he didn't play with it, but held it in his hand, kissed it and at night – placed it under his chin and slept peacefully). Gnome was a vital part of his life that brought feeling of being protected to my boy. When we went on holidays abroad, Gnome was the first to be put into the suitcase (but still the anxious question from Alyosha – 'Have you packed my Gnome yet?' – was asked several times – just to be sure that his little companion wouldn't be left behind).

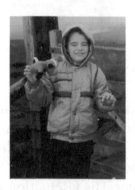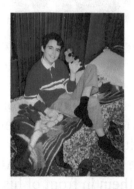

'Gnome, the traveller. Two countries, 5 years in-between – Gnome was always there.'

Favourites change: Elephant to the Rescue

Alas, after hundreds of times going through the washing machine, dozens of patches, stiches and several attempts of restoration, Gnome has now retired to the shelf in Alyosha's bedroom. For the last few decades, his favourites are toy elephants (he possesses a collection of them – from different countries – but only two or three are in 'active service'): he chooses which one goes on holiday or to the respite care.

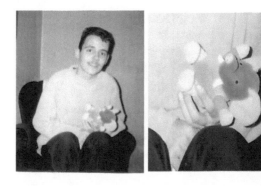

'One of the Gnome's successors in active service'

As Alyosha is an adult now, the question arises: Is it age appropriate? – No, it isn't. But do I care? Let me show you my logic: the first thing to do is to find a mirror, and (while looking at yourself) think very carefully: do 'normal' people always engage in logical (and age-appropriate) activities? I don't think so. For the life of me I can't understand what's so enjoyable, meaningful (and age-appropriate) to watch grown-up (!) men running around one ball? Give them a ball each and let them play! However, despite my reservations, I don't object to my partner watching football matches on TV (and sometimes behaving like a child – shouting and cheering). Why can't we respect autistic people's choices instead of judging them as 'inappropriate'?

The elephants do not embarrass Alyosha – he doesn't see them as toys but rather treats them as companions who help him feel safe in unfamiliar (and constantly changing) environments.

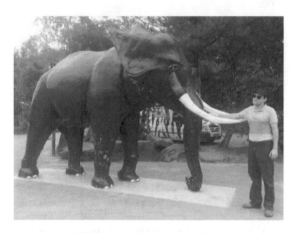

'We find elephants everywhere'

7

—.—

FIVE POLICEMEN, ONE DISLOCATED SHOULDER AND A VERY UPSET CHILD

When Alyosha hit puberty (at 11 and a half years of age), it was nearly impossible to take him out anywhere – he was easily overloaded in situations which, for us, are 'normal' (in supermarkets or other crowded places).

Alyosha was twelve, when we decided to go to Amsterdam – for the first time. As it was just for a weekend, we carefully planned the visit – to see as much as possible and (as it's often the case) saw very little (nothing, to be exact). The most memorable event there, was our close encounter with the Dutch police. (And the only thing I can say about those five police officers is how impressed I was with their professionalism and understanding.)

We started our sightseeing trip from the main square of the city. Though objectively unfair, I blamed the sun for what happened there (I just had to find a culprit) that effectively cut our acquaintance with the city of tulips short. The weather was wonderful! Bright sunshine, clear sky and a gentle breeze from the river. Great? Not really.

It did not only create a visually disturbing environment for my boy (the sun reflected in the water, creating bright kaleidoscopic images) but it also attracted hundreds and hundreds of families to the centre (adding a lot of chaotic movement and all sorts of noise to the visual distortions).

We were sitting in a café outside by a canal, when Alyosha started twitching his whole body, waving his hands in front of his face. In his left hand, he was holding his Gnome that seemed to fail its responsibility to protect the boy from the dangerous world around him. Alyosha appeared to be so angry with his life saviour's failure to provide the feeling of safety that he attempted to throw the poor stuffed fellow into the canal – with me jumping in the air to save the life of his little companion: catching Gnome and providing it asylum in my handbag. Just the thought of the poor thing drowning and never coming back to safely guide us back to England made me accomplish this acrobatic trick. Instead of rounds of applause from the public, unflattering comments from a few adults about my son's behaviour followed. That was it, the boy 'disappeared' (i.e., he was not in control of his actions) and his uncontrolled body reacted with what was seen as aggression – he lashed out at the nearest person (who happened to stand just behind his chair, taking pictures of the canal).

I don't recommend to follow my example but in situations like this, my strategy is to redirect my son's 'aggression' to myself. Two reasons: 1) My boy looks 'normal' and the people around him don't expect (and are not prepared to) his reactions (misinterpreted as 'aggression'); 2) I know how he'd act and I'm prepared to all his kicks, head butting and hitting.

So I placed myself between Alyosha and the person who'd become his target and tried to shift the focus of his attention to myself, but this time it didn't work. People circled us – the worst they could do under the circumstances – as their curiosity aggravated the situation. While desperately attempting to block Alyosha's uncontrolled hitting, I noticed five (!) police officers running to the scene. So I shouted: 'Please, don't interfere! The boy is autistic. He's experiencing a panic attack. I'm his mother, I'll deal with it.' They stopped but surrounded us, thus creating a shield between the public (who were not in a hurry to leave the 'spectacle') and my son and me. My performance was not very good and in a few minutes, I heard: 'Madam, let us interfere. We won't hurt the boy, we just want to help you.' I accepted the offer and stepped back because the whole situation was going from bad to worse.

The police were very professional: they restricted his movements: with one officer on the ground holding his legs, and the rest dealing with the upper part of the panicking body. And very soon my son, with his head sticking out from under the policeman's arm, uttered: 'Help! I'm stuck.' He sounded exhausted.

The end was very emotional. We both were crying – relieved that the nightmare was over. Yes, there were losses (my dislocated shoulder, mild concussion and a couple of bruises), but I couldn't blame my son – he was devastated and remorseful ('I didn't want to hurt you. I won't do it again, I'll fight my panic.' – he was sincere, even if he won't be able to keep his promise in some situations.) In fact, it was me who (unintentionally) exposed him to the situation he couldn't cope with. I felt how unfair it was for my boy who suffered because I couldn't protect him.

This incident made me seek medical help for myself and my son. Before our 'sightseeing in Amsterdam', I was against any medication. I've seen people on huge doses – who were quiet, but not 'here' – 'absent' from what's going on around them, i.e., it was done for carers/teachers, not for the individuals. It was reading the personal accounts by two people I trust (Donna Williams and Temple Grandin) that persuaded me to try a medical route. Both authors emphasised that during puberty, medication (different for each of them) helped them enormously. However, the dose should be the smallest dose possible.

Back home, we booked an appointment with a child psychiatrist, and by trial and error, found the best medication (in the smallest dose possible) for my son.

* * * * *

 ## Notes in the Margin – The causes of sensory overload

The causes of information overload can be: the inability to filter out irrelevant or excessive information; delayed processing; if the person works in mono but is forced to attend to the information from several sensory channels simultaneously; hypersensitivity; distorted or fragmented perception, anxiety, confusion, frustration and stress that, in turn, may lead to challenging behaviour. Each individual may cope with overwhelming stimuli in different ways: mono-processing, avoidance of direct perception, withdrawal, stereotypies.

 ## There's always a BUT – Coping Strategies: Shutdowns

Autistic children learn very early in life to control their environment and the amount of information coming in. To avoid painful sounds, they shut down hearing (though certain frequencies cannot be shut down). Continuous noises (fans, microwave, heating) that don't bother other people may be very annoying. Many children are suspected to be deaf, as they sometimes don't react to sounds. This was a common scene in our household when Alyosha was a toddler, I called out or even shouted my son's name (who was in the same room) and... no reaction whatsoever (not even a blink) from him, as if the boy was deaf. At one occasion a nurse was present and swiftly made some notes on his medical card, then turned to me to say that she'd refer him to a specialist to check his hearing. I knew it would be a useless exercise as his hearing was more acute than 'normal': when I unwrapped his favourite biscuits in the kitchen, Alyosha was next to me in seconds. When the sensory input became too intense and painful, the boy learned to switch off his hearing and withdraw into his own world.

During sensory overload the child can lose some or all of the normal functioning. Systems shutdowns are an involuntary adaptation when the brain turns certain systems off to improve the level of functioning in others.

The process from sensory overload to systems shutdowns may be fast (i.e., sensory discomfort may be short lasting or not experienced at all) or may be slow (i.e., sensory torture may be prolonged). To switch off the painful channel, they may engage in stereotypic behaviours, or deliberately distract themselves through other senses (for example, touching objects when vision or hearing is overwhelming), or withdraw altogether.

If they learn to shut down their systems early in life, they create self-imposed sensory deprivation – thus missing out in development of social and communication skills and experiences of 'normal' ways of functioning.

 ## Do's and Dont's – Protecting from sensory overload

Many autistic children are very vulnerable to sensory overload - the overload comes when they have taken in more than they can keep up with.

Learning to recognise sensory overload is very important. It is better to prevent it than to deal with the consequences. A child vulnerable to sensory overload needs to be in control of his/her environment. Learning to recognize early signs of coming sensory overload is very important. A child may need a quiet place (the 'isle of safety') to recover, where he can go to 'recharge his batteries' from time to time. Stay calm – your nervousness will only add to the child's stress and overload. Never shout, keep any verbal explanation to the minimum. You can discuss the accident later, when the child has calmed down.

As soon as you notice early signs of coming sensory overload (which are different for different individuals), stop the activity and provide time and space to recover, for example, invite the child to get into a quiet place or outside. A 'First Aid Kit' (for sensory overload) should be always at hand. Possible contents may include: sunglasses, ear plugs, squeezy toys, favourite objects and 'I need help' card. When overloaded, even high-functioning autistic children can (temporarily) lose their ability to talk, so the card, which they have been taught to give to the adult present can be very useful.

It is also necessary to teach the individual how to recognise the internal signs of the overload (you cannot be with your child all the time) and ask for help or use different strategies (for example, relaxation techniques) to prevent the problem.

These children have no control over their problems, as they are caused by neurological differences.

The environment may either speed up the development or hinder it. For example, there are many challenging behaviours (for instance, self-injury or meltdowns) that can be dealt with effectively by simply changing the environment. It is impossible for these children to learn if they are bombarded with sensory stimuli coming from all directions. Is it any wonder that they are likely to display behavioural problems, such as self-stimulation, self-injury, aggression, avoidance, rigidity, high anxiety or panic attacks?

Many behaviours that interfere with learning and social interaction are, in fact, protective or sensory defensive responses of the person to 'sensory pollution' in the environment. So, what can you do?

· Always warn the child about the possibility of the stimulus he/she is fearful of and show the source of it. Often it is not the stimulus itself that can trigger what we call difficult/ challenging behaviours, but rather the inability to control or predict it.
· Regular physical exercises are very helpful to decrease stress and calm the child.
· If nothing else works – consider medication (especially, in puberty). Consult a specialist to select the right medication and dose for the child.

 ## Pause for Thought – One sense at a time

Most people use their senses simultaneously, so when they are listening to something, they are still aware of what they see and feel emotionally and physically but some autistic individuals (who are unable to filter incoming information) find it hard (if not impossible) to process information coming in from all the senses, so they often switch to monoprocessing – using one sensory channel at a time. The term (and the concept) of 'monoprocessing'

was introduced by Donna Williams: All channels but one are 'on hold'. It is one thing to *perceive* (at the stage of sensation), but to process all this information is a different matter altogether. If you are not sure what it is or which channel 'is on' at the moment (in the case of fluctuation), use multi-sensory presentation and watch which sensory modality 'is open'. (Remember though that they can switch channels.)

To avoid sensory overload, only one modality is processed consciously by the brain. The child focuses on seeing something but doesn't understand what he's told and doesn't feel being touched or what he/she thinks or feels about the touch. To process the location or special significance of being touched while someone is showing them something means that they see nothing but meaningless colour, and form, and movement.

If the child's vision is unreliable (fragmented or distorted), he/she can focus on the sound, for example, but then the sound may be experienced louder because it is all the child is focusing on. It can lead to hypersensitivity of the only 'active' sensory channel, so they might touch something and send the information through a different sensory channel, thus getting a break for their 'overworked' sense. Switching between the channels gives them an opportunity to be aware, though partially, of what is going on around them, through the sensory modality available to them at the moment.

Or take another example: an autistic student cannot take notes at the lecture because he can either listen or write, but not both. Some of his teachers might think he is being lazy or inattentive because he doesn't look at his teacher, just sitting there with a blank look on his face, but, in fact, he is just focusing on what his lecturer is saying. He is very good at doing one thing at a time.

Actually, this type of processing is taken advantage of by some parents of autistic children who are 'picky-eaters'. Children with very restricted diets (hypersensitive to taste/smell, texture of the food) will eat better if they are watching a video, listening to music or talking to someone.

If the child works in 'mono', it's useful to reduce all irrelevant multisensory stimulation and present information to the child through the sense which is 'on' at the moment. For example, Sasha, a 7-year-old (non-verbal) autistic boy has learned many skills (including reading – with plastic or wooden letters) through touch, with his eyes firmly closed during the process.

We should be aware of this style of perception in order to give the child information in a way he will be able to process. The matter is complicated by the fact, that they could switch channels and our task is to find out which channel 'is open' to get the information.

A child with mono-processing may have problems with multiple stimuli.

How to help:

· Find out which channel 'is open' at the moment.

· Always present information in the child's preferred modality.

· If you are not sure what it is or which channel 'is on' at the moment(in the case of fluctuation), use multi-sensory presentation and watch which sensorymodality 'is open'. (Remember though that they can switch channels.)

8

NOT SUCH A BONDING EXPERIENCE

In many books about autism, there are sections on 'challenging behaviour'. It's understandable as self-injury, running away, hitting, kicking and other difficult behaviours – all can be a part of the condition that has to be dealt with for the sake of both the child and those around him/her. However, the way such behaviours are interpreted is often misleading.

I've read reports about my son's behaviour at school and in many of them there were descriptions of his "aggressive outbursts". Yes, on the surface he seemed aggressive – lashing out at people or attacking the furniture, - but he was actually suffering as much as his 'victim'. After such 'incidents' ("aggression" in reports), he cried and apologised ('I didn't want to hurt you') and I knew he was telling the truth; he had no intention to harm anyone. His 'aggression' indicated that he was not coping and was not in control of his actions.

Here is a paradox: so-called 'aggressive' or 'violent' behaviour can often be a positive sign. It shows that these children *want* (and do their best) to be with us. These 'difficult' children are doing their best *to reach us, to communicate with us.*

Those who work with so-called 'aloof' or 'withdrawn' children know how hard it is to reach them and involve them in any activity. These children seem very happy in their own world and are not motivated to reach out. In contrast, those whom we call 'challenging' (and even aggressive or violent) are *highly* motivated to be part of society.

As one of my friends with autism (in reports, described as 'prone to aggression') says, "I've always wanted to fit in, to *belong* to my family, to our community, to the mainstream society. I wanted to do everything others did, despite my restrictions [being easily overloaded in crowded places and intolerant to noise and the sounds others seem to be ignorant of]. Well, in many cases it didn't work. It's very frustrating."

I can relate to that, as I see how desperately my son wants to participate in whatever we do as a family. To help him, I started a desensitisation programme when he was very young – exposing him to many experiences in small doses, giving him power to control his environment, that is, how much of the stimulation he could cope with and how long he could tolerate it for. It worked, and in a few years, we were able to go to many different places and enjoy many activities together.

However, I've made a few (okay, quite a few) mistakes along the way. For example, after he'd enjoyed 'Harry Potter and Philosopher's Stone' at the cinema (quite a long film), we decided to go and see the last James Bond film with Pierce Brosnan – a decision I regretted 40 minutes into the film. The sound was too loud, there were flashing images on the screen, people crunching popcorn in the seats next to ours... I saw my boy wasn't coping: he started kicking the seat in front of him and shouting 'Stop it!'

He needed to get out as soon as possible but my suggestion to leave was met with loud protestations: "No, no, no! I want to watch it. We are a family!" The situation went from bad to worse with help from the audience. There were two battles going on here – one between James Bond and the bad guy; and the other, between me and my son. For some reason, people in the cinema were much more interested in the outcome of the latter (perhaps because they were sure that Bond would win anyway).

I tried to persuade Alyosha to leave the cinema by promising everything under the sun (starting with ice cream and ending with a trip to Mars) while attempting to minimise the damage caused by his 'aggression'. Eventually, I succeeded. Once we were outside the building, we both were crying: my son sobbing with remorse and me telling him that it's not his fault and that I know what's happened.

It is important to remember, that when an autistic child exhibits what looks like aggression, it does not necessarily mean that it's malicious behaviour. Often it just shows that the child is not coping and is not in control of his actions.

P.S. Oh, and I don't remember the name of the film – as the experience was too traumatic. (Whenever it is on TV now, I always switch to a different channel).

* * * * *

 ## Notes in the Margin – The ABC Approach

When we come across a behaviour that's difficult, there's a popular method that's used to help parents and carers to analyse what's happening and do something about it. You may have heard about it – or even used it. It's called the ABC approach, which stands for Antecedent, Behaviour and Consequence.

Using this approach, the idea is that you find a trigger for the behaviour (Antecedent), define the Behaviour and provide the 'Consequence' for this (often deemed 'inappropriate') behaviour.

 ## There's always a BUT – It is not as simple as ABC

To find a trigger is not as simple as ABC. From my experience, in autism this approach doesn't always work for a number of reasons. Sometimes the antecedent cannot be easily identified. Let me explain.

Present but invisible antecedent
Sometimes we cannot see/hear/feel certain stimuli as our senses are too 'normal'. For example, the child may

be disturbed by the sound of the microwave oven two rooms away. You may not be able to hear it yourself, so any 'challenging behaviour' might look as if it's come 'out of the blue'.

Possible future antecedents

How do you identify an antecedent when it hasn't happened yet? Since any sudden unpredictable stimuli (such as a noise, for example) can be painful to a child with autism, sometimes it's fear alone that can cause a behaviour, in anticipation of something unpleasant.

There are a multitude of environmental threats like this - school bells, fire alarms, fans, dogs barking and vacuum cleaners are all common ones. So, always warn a child about the possibility of the noise they are fearful of and show where it is coming from. Showing them a hairdryer or vacuum cleaner for a few minutes and letting them control the switch themselves is one way to help.

Past antecedent

Sometimes any stimuli (not only sensory but also emotional ones) may be associated with painful memories of pain, anger, or panic. As any memory brought to the surface becomes very much *present*, the child may react in the way they reacted in the past when the bad experience happened for real.

What can provoke anger, fear, anxiety or a panic attack? Anything! From smell to what can be called 'emotionally coloured intonations'. For example, some smells can bring pleasurable memories and other odours remind children of unhappy ones – and some words have 'emotional colouring' that can be negatively charged. In autism, the conventional interpretation often doesn't matter. If something unpleasant happened when the child heard the word 'sorry', for example, they would connect this word with the experience. Any time the child hears 'Sorry!' he may react with rage – the experience repeats itself.

The 'last straw' antecedent

Sometimes there are no definite triggers whatsoever! The cause of the 'challenging' behaviour may simply be overload. So, if your child has been struggling already, anything can be the 'last straw'.

The emotional state of the carer/teacher as an antecedent

As most autistic children's senses work in 'hyper', and feelings start as sensations (either conscious or unconscious), it is no wonder that many autistic people are emotionally hypersensitive, too. Some resonate with the emotional states of those around them.

Sometimes the carers themselves (or rather their emotional states) trigger the challenging behaviours in these children. They may feel the negative emotions of their carers but cannot interpret what (and why) they are feeling.

If you feel under the weather, don't think that you can pretend everything is fine and the children won't notice. They won't understand what's wrong but they will *sense* the negative signals you're emitting (at a subliminal level – resonance*/ echoemotica*).

Some synaesthetic experiences (see chapter 11).

Do's and Dont's

As the children are unable to cope with the demands of the world they are not equipped to deal with, they are likely to display behavioural problems, such as self-stimulation, self-injury, aggression, avoidance, rigidity, high anxiety, panic attacks, etc. It is important to remember that these children have no control over their problems, as they are caused by neurological differences. 'Rewards' and 'punishments' (to manipulate triggers and/or consequences of the behaviour) are useless at best and cruel at worst.

Autistic children are often engaged in stereotyped activities/behaviours – often called *stimming** – such as rocking, spinning, flapping their hands, tapping things, watching things spin, etc.

We can get a lot of information from observing the child's stims. These (typical in autism) behaviours are often called 'bizarre' or 'abnormal', while, in fact, they're compensatory strategies the child has acquired to regulate their sensory systems and cope with 'unwelcome stimulation' or lack of it. That's why no matter how irritating and meaningless these behaviours may seem to us, it is unwise to stop them without learning the function they serve and introducing experiences with the same function. Repetitive behaviours in ASD may serve several different purposes. These may be:

- Defensive: in order to reduce the pain or discomfort caused by hypersensitivities, overload, etc.

- Self-stimulatory: to improve the input, for example, in the case of hyposensitivity
- Compensatory: to interpret the environment in the case of unreliable sensory information (fragmentation, distortions, sensory agnosia*)
- Out of frustration
- Just pleasurable experiences that help to withdraw from a confusing and/or overwhelming environment.

Simple? Not really, because one and the same behaviour may have different underlying causes, requiring different treatment/support. For example, a boy flaps his hand in front of his face can mean that the child has (hyper) painful visual experiences, or he can have (hypo) vision and tries to stimulate it, or to ignore 'offending' and confusing stimuli around him.

If you try to eliminate a behavior without having found the function of it, the child will have to replace it with another one (with the same function) and the 'replacement' will not necessarily be a better one.

So don't aim to eliminate the child's stims (no matter how annoying they are) but rather replace them with 'more acceptable ones' with the same function. For instance, if the child chews his clothes, give him something else to chew. With development, some behaviours will disappear, while some others will be replaced by other behaviours.

Alyosha used to run in circles, jump up and down, or just sit quietly, flapping a toy (actually – anything would do – including his hand or fingers – for this activity) in front of his eyes. Or, he would be scratching the surface of his coloured blocks, or turning the wheels of his toy car, or slamming feet or just banging doors for hours. These behaviours increased when the boy was anxious – helping to decrease stress, or when he was bored. When Alyosha was engaged in something, stimming decreased. Hence whenever possible, I involved him in all sorts of activities.

The irony was that my misfortune (I was a single mother in a foreign country without any support from the state) turned into an advantage for Alyosha: Whilst he was a child, I had to take him everywhere with me (if I couldn't find a baby-sitter) – to lectures and seminars at university or even to important social engagements (where I worked as an interpreter). From a very early age, Alyosha 'attended' many VIP social events in many different venues (including posh restaurants), and public celebrations. I did my best to help him cope and at the same time, not to embarrass my little gentleman and let him enjoy himself.

For example, one evening, after a dinner in a restaurant with VIPs, the guests started dancing. Alyosha got up, went to the centre of the room (he loved the music) and also started 'dancing' (moving from one foot to the other while rocking his body). I positioned myself in front of him and started dancing (slightly imitating his movements but giving them a 'social touch') – as if we were performing in a dancing competition (later I watched *Strictly Come Dancing* and immediately recognised myself as a 'professional dancer' with Alyosha as a 'celebrity'.) I heard one of the puzzled VIPs, saying to his partner: "You said the child was abnormal, but look how well he's dancing with his mother. I like his very original moves..."

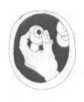 **Pause for Thought – Aisle Be Back (Why We Steered Clear from the Supermarket...)**

Having trouble shopping with an autistic youngster? I understand this problem only too well; from the time my son was a toddler, it was impossible to take him shopping with me. Anything (and I do mean ANYTHING) could trigger his meltdown. Sometimes I could identify the cause of it (even if it took days after the event) – constantly playing the 'video' of the latest catastrophe in my head until I found a more or less rational explanation. My boy was bombarded with noises from all directions, drowned in lights, attacked by smells and disoriented by people moving in chaotic patterns. His tinted glasses helped but it was not enough. We can't adjust all the places to his needs. For example, I couldn't enter whatever supermarket we opted to visit beforehand demanding all the lights were switched off, whilst escorting all mothers with young children out and ordering the rest to move one by one in a straight line, keeping their voices down (or even not talking at all while my son was at the premises)? The solution was to desensitise him to different places and situations. We started with shopping.

Operation 'Supermarket' was likely to be long-term and needed a lot of planning and organisation. We decided that every Sunday morning we'd go shopping in a big supermarket (the same supermarket at the first stage of the adventure), equipped with tinted glasses and ear-defenders against the visual and auditory 'offences'.

Starting with small doses of the shopping experience, we hoped to desensitise my boy's ability to tolerate the stimuli that other people were comfortable with.

The first time was the most successful. However, it was too early to celebrate. Yes, Alyosha did cope with his first visit of the supermarket, but his 'stay' there lasted all of 30 seconds. We went in with a trolley (and determination) yet had to leave pretty soon afterwards. Still, it was a start!

The week after, we managed to reach the first aisle and spent nearly two minutes inside. The following weeks, our shopping experience lasted longer and longer and longer and I realised he was finally beginning to get accustomed to the foreign nature of the place and the stimuli.

Fast forward a year: our shopping trips were no problem (not only in this supermarket but at any other shop). Alyosha happily pushed the trolley, zigzagging along the aisles, correcting 'the wrongs' on his way (picking up misplaced things and putting them where they should be, straightening the rows of tins and cans, etc).

From time to time, there were moments when my interference was necessary – for such situations we'd developed a scenario to help him relax and focus on his duties. So, if he heard a baby crying far away from us at the other end of the supermarket, he looked at me and officially announced: 'A baby is crying,' expecting me to say my lines of our pre-approved 'play script'. (This was not the time to develop flexibility). I always obliged: 'Yes, the baby is crying because it's small and stupid. You are big and clever, so you behave like an adult.' Anyone could see that Alyosha felt much better and was doing his best not to react to the painful sound. But that wasn't all, as I always added, 'When you were a baby you also cried but now you've grown up.'

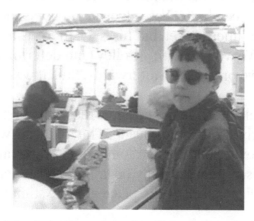

'Alyosha had become comfortable in supermarkets.'

Has it been always 'happily ever after'? Not quite. For example, to take him pre-Christmas shopping in an unfamiliar supermarket (about 18 years ago) was a big mistake. Our usual shopping adventure turned into a nightmare.

There were HUNDREDS of people in the supermarket; music, sales announcements, babies crying, people talking and moving in all directions, long queues... In 15 minutes, I could see that the overload was setting in. My boy was feeling attacked and I could see he was in pain. The last straw was when a lady tried to reach the shelf from behind while we were standing in a queue. Alyosha lashed out at her. I attempted to get him out as soon as possible but all the aisles were blocked by trolleys and people. Those around us were staring (and it did not help as Alyosha could not tolerate any direct perception). While I was dragging him out of the shop, he was kicking the trolleys, pushing people...

Outside my boy was crying, trying to explain: "It was a panic attack. My eyes hurt. I didn't want to hurt anyone. I won't do it again. I will fight my panic." I knew he was doing his best and told him that I understood what had happened, that it was not his fault, that I loved him...

Of course, the people around us had no idea why a handsome teenager was screaming like a baby and being aggressive to others; and his mother, instead of imposing some discipline, was saying how much she loved him... Oh, well...

In this way, I've learnt not to push it too far. But on the whole, Operation Supermarket has been a huge success.

9
—.—

LOOK AT ME WHEN I'M TALKING TO YOU! OR...BETTER, DON'T!

How often do teachers and parents say to a child 'Look at me when I'm talking to you!'? We want the child to pay attention to what we're saying and assume that our (ill-informed) instruction will make them more attentive. How else can we teach our offspring useful skills and provide them with valuable information if their eyes are looking not at us but, say, at the wall or at their feet? This is an absolutely correct approach when we deal with non-autistic children, but when we interact with our autistic kids, insistence on eye contact is likely to confuse them and hinder understanding of what we are trying to inform them about.

I witnessed how one autistic adult, when introduced to a journalist, instead of the meaningless but conventional 'How do you do?' helpfully enquired: 'Do you want eye contact or a conversation?' This response reflects one of the main features of autism – avoidance of direct perception for autistic individuals is another involuntary adaptation that helps them survive in a sensory distorted world by avoiding(or decreasing) information overload.

Autistic children often seem to look past things and seem to be completely 'absent' from the scene. It is their attempt to avoid experiencing a visual/auditory stimulus directly. This strategy gives them the ability to take in sensory information with meaning. They can often understand things better by attending to them indirectly, for example, by looking or listening peripherally (such as out of the corner of one's eye or by looking at or listening to something else). Donna Williams calls it a kind of indirectly confrontational approach in contrast to the 'normal' directly confrontational one.

Some autistic children (and adults) are very hypersensitive when they are approached directly by other people. For some, if they are looked at directly (even if they do not 'return the gaze'), they may feel it on the body – sort of 'distance touching' with actual tactile experience that can be painful. For instance, my son cannot tolerate it when someone is looking at him directly and makes them turn away ('Don't look!' 'Turn away!').

Looking directly at people, or even animals, is too overwhelming. For example, Alyosha complained when our cat looked at him! They say that cats don't like when people look them in the eye – they interpret it as aggression from the humans. And this is true about our cat Dasha. But (perhaps because she's often bored, Dasha's come up with a very funny way to entertain herself) she would sit in front of the boy, while he was watching TV, to look intensely at him. The first time it happened, Alyosha was devastated – he started shouting: "Dasha is looking at me. Tell her to turn away!" I rushed into the living room to see what this commotion was about – to find him with his face covered with his hands, while our feline member of the family sitting in front of him with an innocent look on her furry face. Naively, I thought it'd be easy to stop the turmoil, but, boy, how wrong I was! Just pushing Dasha from her strategically chosen position didn't work – she didn't even blink and remained motionless. Neither was there any reaction to my (angry) voice and my eloquent (not necessarily politically correct) verbal persuasion. With all the diplomatic options exhausted, I turned to sheer force and removed the outraged Dasha from the room.

After this performance had been repeated countless times, turning into a routine – it became clear that Dasha did it deliberately: whenever she wanted some amusement, off she went to find my son and gleefully placed herself the way she could to get his full attention.

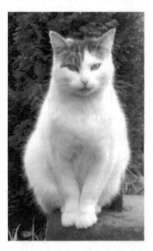

'Dasha seemed to think that her mission was to teach Alyosha eye contact.'
* * * * *

Notes in the Margin – Avoidance of eye contact

Avoidance of eye contact is quite common in autism. One of the explanations for this is that people with autism use peripheral vision because their central vision is hypo- while their peripheral vision is hyper-. In fact, the opposite is much more common: they do not use their direct/central perception because 'it hurts', or is stressful (i.e., it is hyper-). However, some of the problems autistic people have with making eye contact may be nothing more than intolerance for the movement of the other person's eyes.

It turns out that avoidance of direct perception is not restricted only to vision but also includes other sensory systems such as, for example, auditory and tactile. Perceiving sounds, visual stimuli, or touch directly and consciously may often result in fragmentation: the person can interpret the part but lose the whole, and incoming information is interpreted piece by piece.

Direct perception in autism is often hyper. It can cause sensory overload resulting in switching to mono: they actually 'hear better' (i.e., understand what's being said) when they are not looking at the person. They often use their peripheral vision and seem to see what is going on without directly looking at it. The same is true for other senses if they are hypersensitive: indirect perception of smell or 'instrumental touch' are often defensive mechanisms to avoid overload.

There's always a BUT – There is 'eye contact' and eye contact

There is 'eye contact' and eye contact: a child can turn your head and look directly into your eyes – but this has nothing to do with eye contact, it's sensory fascination, which many children enjoy. Eye contact, on the other hand, is looking at the person while talking to him/her, and here we have a problem: direct perception hurts and may result in fragmentation and losing the ability to talk with meaning.

Do's and Dont's

· Never force eye contact. If we want to develop their conversational skills, it's better to forget about eye contact (at least, in the beginning).

Use an indirectly confrontational approach, especially involving hypersensitive modalities. In fact, they understand you better when you do NOT insist on eye contact and talk... to the wall. If you start your lesson, or any other interaction with 'Look at me!' the information will be lost, whereas if you sit next to the child and address all your explanations to the object in front of you both, the child is likely to get the meaning from the situation.

· Do not approach the child directly in his/her hypersensitive modalities.

· When hypersensitivity of the affected sensory channel is addressed and lessened, direct perception becomes easier.

Of course, it is important to teach our children to look at people (or, at least in the direction of the people) when they are talking to them, but it should be gradual with simultaneous work of desensitisation. As they cannot maintain eye contact, teach them to look at the space in between the eyes or at the forehead. To the other person, it looks like you're directly looking at their eyes when, in fact, you're looking in-between. Cheating? Yes, but this strategy helps the child process what his/her communication partner is saying.

Pause for Thought – Face Blindness

There is another neurological condition that, though not specific to autism, appears to be quite common in (at least some) autistic individuals. It's called prosopagnosia, or face blindness. People suffering from this condition have trouble recognizing people's faces. It may be genetic and runs in families (developmental prosopagnosia: at least one first-degree relative, for example, a parent or a sibling has it as well), or it may be caused by strokes, head injuries, or severe illnesses (acquired prosopagnosia). The exact effects and severity may vary between people: some may be blind to all but the most familiar faces, while others (with severe prosopagnosia) cannot recognise even themselves in the mirror. Can you imagine how embarrassing it is when someone (trying to be sociable at a party) cheerfully waves her hand to her own reflection in the mirror?

Non-autistic prosopagnostics say that face blindness tends to isolate them from people in general, as being unable to recognize others interferes with making and maintaining relationships. They work out their own recognition system. Most common features that seem to work best for face blind people are casual clothes, movement, long hair and facial hair (as the inability to recognize faces does not extend to hair, particularly if it is long enough to extend out of the face area). They can see a pattern in hair texture and process hairlines. Interestingly, many autistic children are fascinated by people's hair, and many do not recognize their relatives if they wear unfamiliar clothes.

Another problem prosopagnostic people experience is the difficulty to understand and express emotions. The main 'tools' to express emotions are not words but facial expressions, gestures and tone of voice. For people who cannot 'read' faces because of face blindness or/and cannot 'hear' emotions in voices because of their auditory processing problems, it is extremely difficult not only to understand emotions in others but also to express emotions themselves otherwise than using words. It's sort of 'emotion blindness'. There is a striking similarity of emotional expressions of blind people and individuals with prosopagnosia: not seeing what emotions are supposed to look like when coming in, both the blind and prosopagnostics have never acquired a large repertoire of emotions to send out. It is no wonder, therefore, that autistic people experiencing all sorts of sensory processing problems find it most difficult to understand (conventionally expressed) emotional states of other people and those of their own. (However, autistic individuals often *sense* emotions of others in their own bodies – resonance*/echoemotica* – without interpretation what they mean.)

In addition to their difficulties in 'reading' facial expressions, some prosopagnostic people have problems with understanding gestures and sign language, which involves a lot of facial expressions.

Face blindness may co-occur with autism. Some researchers even suggest that prosopagnosia may be an essential symptom in autistic spectrum disorder, perhaps a specific subgroup of Asperger syndrome. A teenager with Asperger Syndrome often got into embarrassing situations because she did not remember faces unless she had seen the people many times or they had a very distinct facial feature, such as a big beard, thick glasses or a strange hairstyle. A prosopagnostic autistic boy, despite knowing the names of his classmates, often calls them 'a boy' or 'a girl'. Interestingly, when one of the girls had her hair cut short, he 'moved' her to the 'boy' category.

Some experimental studies of autistic people's capacity to process faces suggest that they use abnormal processing strategies and experience less difficulties when faces are presented to them upside-down.

10

— · —

ADVENTURES (AND BATTLES) WITH FOOD

'W e are what we eat' – is a widely accepted statement, and most people do try to eat healthy foods to improve their well-being. However, if we deal with autistic children, there are many problems related to 'healthy food', 'balanced diet' and eating in general. Some will eat anything and everything, whether it is edible or inedible (pica). Others will refuse to eat 99% of the food we offer, and the one per cent they do accept can be the 'wrong' food for them – causing allergies, 'leaky gut syndrome', and which may result in challenging behaviours. For some, food can be a source of fear. Others will accept their 'selected food' only if it is presented the 'right' way, be of the 'right' colour, and of the 'right' shape. If there is the slightest 'fault', they reject it immediately and will go without any food for hours, if not days. Many will refuse to try any new food and keep eating three or four items from the menu for years.

Before we can be sure that we fulfil the nutritional requirements of growing children, we have to make sure that our 'healthy nutritional diet' (with the correct proportions of proteins, fats, carbohydrates, minerals and vitamins) will get into their mouth. And this is a big problem for some autistic children. All the many behavioural suggestions (for example, to encourage your child to try new food, rewarding with stickers) are often inapplicable to some children with autism because they are hypersensitive to certain foods/smells. And there may be more reasons for resistance to some dishes and drinks.

Feeding problems can start from birth (when a baby is very difficult at feeding times), or later. Some children will start off eating everything they are offered but then regress, usually at about 18-24 months. These children limit their total food intake to three or four items (for example, potatoes, pasta, apples) and refuse to try anything from 'outside of their menu'.

Alyosha has always had food issues: for the first three months of his life, my baby was losing weight – constant diarrhea – nothing was held in his stomach. After that an opposite problem arose – chronic constipation. The yo-yo pattern (diarrhea – constipation) continued for years. For the first year, he was a very poor eater, often falling asleep at my breast. With solid food the situation was better but the list of what he was prepared to eat was very limited. Interestingly, at the age of three years, my boy put himself on a partial casein-free diet – he refused point blank to drink milk, while ice-cream was allowed to stay on his menu.

My main concern was the lack of variety of what he accepted at meal times. For the first six years, he ate the same food every day: apples (peeled and cut into quarters with the core removed), pasta and biscuits. His doctor (and my friends) suggested: if he didn't eat what was offered, let him go hungry. A sound advice, wasn't it? It turned out – it wasn't. Alyosha didn't seem to mind to starve himself and happily went without any food for a day. I had to accept that I lost this battle. I skipped plan B (behavioural approach: encourage the child to try new food, rewarding him with something he likes) because it never worked with him so I moved to plan C.

Armed with scissors, cardboard, glue and old magazines I spent the night designing illustrated menus for my little prince. I was so pleased with the results that I would have patted myself on the back if I could. Unable to sleep, I spent a few hours left before the morning, imagining how I'd show my boy the way to choose the food he would like for his breakfast, giving him the power to control what he will consume. Dreams, hopes, optimistic expectations and... a complete failure. Alyosha grabbed a card with a picture of a glass of apple juice (without even looking at the picture) and started flapping it in front of his eyes –laughing happily. (Later I was able to explain his behaviour. His vision was fragmented and unreliable – it wasn't a representation of a glass of juice for him, but a paper card with coloured spots on it – to flap in front of his eyes and to enjoy the sensation.)

What next? Plan D? No, I gave up – at least for that moment – and the boy continued to protest (very loudly) if a new food appeared on his plate – it should be removed. (Even now he doesn't start eating fish and chips if there is a slice of lemon on the plate, or rejects a drink if there are ice cubes in his glass). My reasoning for a break was based

112

on my own experiences. Who was I to insist on him eating the foods he disliked if I've always been picky about what I eat as well? I vividly remember how (when I was about three years old) I (physically) could not eat barley porridge. If encouraged to swallow a spoonful, I 'recycled' it back on the plate as soon as this stuff reached my stomach. Eventually, my parents gave up. The same happened to fried or boiled onion. Having 'food issues' myself, I found it easy to sympathise with Alyosha.

Since the age of 7-8 years, his menu gradually began to expand and in his teen years Alyosha became more adventurous – happy to try new foods: once cheese was unacceptable but now he eats it with pleasure. However, some food is still unacceptable, for example: melons, watermelons, pineapples and tomatoes (strangely, he likes ketchup, though), mushy peas (but he has no problem with green peas).

Did I encourage him to try new foods? Yes, I did, but I never applied any pressure. From experience with autistic children I know – the more you insist, the less likely the child considers to try it. So, these were just (matter-of-factly) suggestions, without any pressure and a look of indifference from me. ('If you don't want it/don't like it – don't eat it' with 'your loss, not mine' attitude.) The less pressure I applied, the keener he was to experiment. Besides, with time (as he became more adventurous), his likes and dislikes changed.

So for my son, the best 'treatment' was time and his increasing awareness of the (social) world around him, his desire to spend more time with us (not just 'physically' being with us, but being one of us – participating in all the family activities). With increased awareness and social experiences, his anxiety lessened and Alyosha's become less rigid about his food. However, his 'eating rituals' are still here: he eats his food in a particular order, one thing at a time (for example, first chips, then fish).

His best incentive is a meal in a restaurant. Perhaps it is not much about the food but rather this is the place where he is allowed a glass of coca-cola on special occasions: Christmas, New Year, birthdays. (The consequences are not good – coca-cola for Alyosha is like alcohol, he becomes very difficult to be with, so the drink appears only at big celebrations.) Talking about alcohol, my son is an adult now, and I did give him wine, beer and champagne to try (watching anxiously for his reaction). And with each of them, his feedback brought relief and peace to my mind: his face wrinkled up into a funny grimace while he uttered his verdict – "Disgusting!"

* * * * *

 Notes in the Margin – Feeding problems

The most obvious 'feeding problems' seem to be related to *taste/smell hypersensitivities*. For some, almost all types of food smell too sharp. Their sense of taste is so acute that if they are offered, for example, something they like (but a recipe has slightly changed) they would not accept it. If a tiny amount of new food is added to the food they like, it will be discarded as inedible.

Children with *hypotaste/hyposmell* chew and smell everything they can get – grass, flowers, dirt, play dough, toothpaste and so on. They sniff and lick objects, play with faeces. (However, not all 'smelling/tasting behaviours' indicate hyposensitivity, sometimes it is the only reliable channel for the children whose visual perception is distorted (unreliable) so they have to smell everything to be sure what is in front of them. When visual problems are addressed, the behaviour disappears.)

What complicates the matter is, that the child's sensitivity can *fluctuate* (from hyper- to normal/ hypo- and vice versa). What was a favourite food for years, one day can become absolutely unacceptable.

In this context, one should mention also *idiosyncratic tastes*: some will eat 'incompatible foods' together, for instance, ice-cream with gherkins.

Apart from the senses of taste and smell, there are other, equally important sensory perceptual issues, which contribute to the eating problems. Thus, other sensory channels' abnormalities can aggravate the situation. For example:

- Some children do not experience hunger (in the case of *hypointeroception*) – their body does not tell them when it is time to eat; they can go without any food for very long periods of time, without being bothered about it, so they have to be reminded of meal times and encouraged to eat something.

-     *Motor problems* are quite common: some children have difficulties swallowing, others have problems with chewing so they swallow everything as a whole.

-       Texture of the food is very important: some children cannot tolerate any (even the tiniest) lumps in their food which should be consistently smooth, others would eat only dry foods with crunchy bits – anything with gravy or sauces is unacceptable. It is not the case of stubbornness, but rather a physical problem of certain *textures intolerance*, when a child becomes sick if the food of the 'wrong' texture gets into his mouth. That is why these children have to touch the food before they eat it; if they do not like the feel of it, they reject it without tasting.

-     Some are very peculiar about the *temperature* of the food: some will eat only cold foods and drink cold drinks.

-     *Auditory and visual* modalities are also involved in the 'assessment' of foods on offer. Thus, the *sound* the food produces in the mouth can be unbearable and frightening. Because of literalness and inability to filter sensory information, appearance is extremely important: the container/package should be the same or the child may reject even his favourite food or drink. The food (that they accept) should come from the same package – with the same picture in front, of the same colour and the same design. The look of the food is very important, too. If something they like looks slightly different or 'imperfect' (for example, toast is not 'brown enough', or there is an eye in a cooked potato) it will be discarded straightaway.

-   The *colour* plays a huge role in acceptance of certain foods. For example, some children would not touch (to say nothing of putting in the mouth) anything red or yellow.

-   Quite a few children would reject even their favourite food if it is of the 'wrong *shape*'.

-   *Presentation* on the plate (and on the table) can create problems as well: some children will refuse to eat if there are different foods on the same plate, or if different foods touch each other as if they become 'contaminated'. Others will re-arrange the food on their plate to be symmetrical before they put it in the mouth.

-   Still some others will eat and drink only from a particular plate or cup, for example, they insist on the 'juice cup' which is different from the 'water cup'; even their favourite food/drink presented on the 'wrong' plate/in the 'wrong' cup will not be touched.

There are many other issues that can affect eating behaviours, most common being:

- The *ritual* is very important for many autistic children: they insist on certain rituals before they eat even their favourite foods, for instance, packages should be open in a certain way, certain foods should be sliced a particular way, etc. A child can eat certain foods at home on a Sunday but refuse to eat the very same food on a Wednesday or in school (because it is 'Sunday food' eaten at home), and vice versa: what is acceptable in school, is out of the question at home.

- The *fear of change*, of anything new and unfamiliar often leads to a strong aversion to eating or drinking anything new and unfamiliar. They would stick with what they know and like, without any desire to add anything new to their menu: they have no need for variety in their food because they like 'sameness' and will eat the same for years.

- Some are fearful of growing up and get very upset about it: they dislike changes in their bodies and reject food in hope that they stay the way they are if they do not eat. On the other hand, some children, if told that this particular food will help them become strong and big, will be motivated to eat it.

- *Favourites*: There are some foods (different for different children) that they crave (and usually the favourite items are not on a 'healthy list of nutritional foods'). Some children dip all the foods they eat into ketchup, or a particular sauce.

 ## There's always a BUT – What causes what?

There are several issues to consider: Is the primary problem sensory perceptual difficulties, which lead to restricted nutritional input? Or is it biochemical abnormalities creating sensory perceptual difficulties? Perhaps, even both?

In some autistic people, sensory problems, such as sensory overload or sensory hypersensitivities may be caused by certain vitamin-mineral deficiencies and food and chemical allergies. It may be possible to address these by exploring underlying biochemical problems, such as hormone imbalances and their effects on enzyme production affecting digestion, the synthesis of vitamins and minerals and their interconnectedness with auto-immune problems such as food and chemical allergies and intolerances. For example, for Donna Williams candida albicans* was one of the major contributors to her sensory perceptual and some other autism-related problems.

On the other hand, some of these metabolic and chemical problems can be due to chronic heightened stress caused by sensory perceptual problems. In this sense, the two can become a vicious circle. For example, vitamin B, magnesium and zinc deficiencies can relate to pitch and brightness hypersensitivity, although whether these vitamins and minerals are consumed in coping with these sensitivities or whether they make a person more vulnerable and susceptible to these hypersensitivities is not clear and only further research can answer that.

Do's and Dont's

Understanding causes of children's food intolerances and idiosyncratic eating behaviours is vital if we want to help them. If we start with addressing diagnostic features of the condition but neglecting the causes of these features (that can be different in different children), any improvements will be unlikely.

119

Some sensory perceptual difficulties can be caused by correctable problems, which, if addressed, can affect the efficiency of functioning through improving the supply of nutrients and reduction of toxicity (for example, treatment of the fungal infection, candida albicans; casein/gluten intolerances, vitamin-mineral/ amino acids problems, etc.). Other problems can include metabolic disorders, 'gut leakages', viral infections, etc. Reduced delivery of nutrients to the brain through the blood can mean limited ability to process information, delayed processing, sensory hypersensitivity, overload and shutdowns.

- Desensitisation techniques address the problems directly: if the child is hypersensitive to touch, facial and oral massage may be used, then gradual desensitisation to textures, sounds, tastes, smells, etc.

- Such behavioural suggestions as to encourage so-called picky eaters to try new food, rewarding them with something they like do not work for many autistic individuals. If children are hypersensitive to certain foods/smells they cannot even stay in the proximity of anyone eating because of the intolerable smell. Some children would vomit if they encounter the smell they cannot tolerate, which they can detect even from two rooms away. Behavioural methods ignore real difficulties some children experience and often create more problems than provide solutions. The more pressure is applied, the stronger the resistance. The extreme form – force-feeding – will make the situation even worse.

- On the other hand, encouragement through fading* while addressing the sensitivity problems and offering rewards with recognition (praise – in a neutral manner!) of the child's efforts to achieve it is a better option and worth trying. Starting with acceptance of a new food on the child's plate, to letting the food to touch face, then lips, to very small amount of the food in the mouth, and finally swallowing it.

- Keeping the pressure off and creating the least fuss about trying new foods will bring better results – the child is more relaxed and may become more curious about new foods that others eat and would want to try. If the new food is regularly presented on the table, the child may get accustomed to the sight, smell and feel of it without any pressure from the parents. Asking (from time to time) if he wants to try it can result one day in 'Yes, please.' Gradual introduction is a slow process but with patience and consistency it works for some children.

- Disguising new food, for example, under ketchup (if the child likes ketchup) may work for some children.

- Providing new foods that look similar to those they already like: some may try something if it looks similar to what they like.

- Structure and routine: creating new routines (introducing new foods in new places, for instance).

- Eating in a new environment can bring both problems and opportunities. For example, the chaos in school at lunchtime and pressure from lunchtime staff can put the child off not only from trying something new but also from eating his/her packed lunch. On the other hand, a thorough preparation and introduction of a new 'eating routine' (which will include new food in the menu) in a new setting can encourage the child to try new food (which will be associated with this place and routine).

- Using visual aids, written rules and social stories explaining what is expected in certain situations may be successful with some children.

- Sometimes offering 'character meals' (food in shapes of characters, objects, etc., the child is interested in) can encourage the child to try new food. But the effect can be the opposite for other children – they can refuse to eat their 'favourite characters'. Favourite characters can also be used as role models, for example, if the child likes rabbits, telling him that his favourite rabbit likes carrots may encourage him to eat it.

- Because many autistic children monoprocess (use only one sensory channel at a time), distraction can be used with them, for example, if they are watching TV or reading a book while eating, they may be unaware of what exactly they are eating or what they think or feel about it. This type of processing is taken advantage of by the parents of some autistic children with very restricted diets who will eat better if they are watching a video, listening to music or talking to someone.

- Some faddy eaters can be encouraged to choose the food they would like to eat (for example, giving them two different options). This will give them some control of the eating process. Yet again, there may be difficulties with this as well: if both options are unacceptable, or difficulties to make a choice, etc.

- In some cases, children become more 'adventurous' if they are involved in the whole process – starting from buying necessary ingredients in the supermarket, opening packets, (if they can tolerate the smell) cooking, serving, and then eating the food.

- Peer pressure and desire to please family is relevant for children with Asperger syndrome who want to fit in and/or to make their parents happy, but it is unlikely to work with someone on the more severe end of the autistic spectrum. Some will agree to try a new food but insist on having a glass of water to wash it down in case they do not like it. Some will listen to explanations about different products and their benefits for the organism and will be eager to eat 'healthy foods'.

- Children with very restricted diets can be given mineral and vitamin supplements.

 ## Pause for Thought – Not Autism, but Autisms

Research into special diets has been criticised for being 'anecdotal' or lacking 'scientific evidence'. However, none of the approaches (sensory treatments, behavioural methods, medications, etc.) would benefit the average person with autism. The reason is that autism is a heterogeneous* condition, i.e., there are numerous underlying causes, for example, genetic, biochemical, structural and functional differences in the brain, environmental or combinations of these, which are different for different people. However, all these causes lead to the same clinical manifestation of the condition. And the outcomes are different for seemingly similar children. Thus, there is no one size fits-all treatment.

In other words, there is no autism, but rather autismS – each caused by different problems in different individuals but leading to the same behaviours 'on the surface', and there may be different types of autism (phenotypes*) in different people and sometimes more than one type of autism present in the same person. That is why what works for some will be useless (or even harmful) to others. The manifestations of sensory perceptual problems are very different in different individuals.

Keeping in mind that there are no two autistic individuals with the exactly same sensory-perceptual profile, specialists working with this population should approach each case individually and decide what is best for each particular child. Sometimes mistakes will be made, but by trial and error (and with consistency and patience) we can change 'what they eat' to make them healthier and happier. The process may be slow and complicated, but let us remember – whatever autism is, it is never boring

11

— · —

THE WORLD WITH AN EXTRA DIMENSION

"Two little eyes to look around.
Two little ears to hear each sound,
One little nose to smell..."

We all know the lines and happily sing them with our children. But what if eyes can see sounds, ears can hear tastes, noses can smell colours? Does it sound absurd? Not for those with cross-sensory perception, the common term for synaesthesia. Synaesthesia is the ability to perceive stimulation of one sensory modality via a different sensory channel. To translate it into plain English: those with synaesthesia see sounds, hear or smell colours, taste shapes, or feel sounds on the skin. Some people may forget the name of the person they know but remember the colour, taste, or even temperature of the word.

Although not specific to autism, synaesthesia seems to be quite common among autistic individuals.

If you can answer questions like these, you have synaesthesia:

Can you see sounds?

Can you taste or hear colours?
Can you feel shapes on your skin when you smell something?
What do sounds taste like?
What colour is Wednesday?

Alyosha was about nine years old when he tried to account for a panic attack by saying: "I was scared. I saw a yellow 'z-z-z' sound." This was confusing, until I realised he had cross-sensory perception.

There are many different types and variations of synaesthesia; for example, according to the number of senses involved there are:

- *two-sensory synaesthesia* (when stimulation of one sense triggers the perception in a second sense). So, someone may complain about the sour taste of the neighbour's voice. There can be many different combinations of senses.

- *multi-sensory synaesthesia* (when more than two senses are involved). That's when it gets really complicated! A child may experience the taste of the sound, while simultaneously seeing the colour and experiencing a tickling sensation on the skin. Examples of seeing colours while hearing sounds in synaesthesia are well known. Some individuals seem to see not only the colours of their acoustic environment but also the density, shape and movement of sounds.

In autism, quite common is the form of synaesthesia that produces tactile sensations without the individual being physically touched, for example, looking at something can bring a tactile experience. Or the other way round, when somebody looks (or stares) at them directly, they

126

feel it on the skin. Some autistic individuals experience 'being touched' by sounds, i.e., certain sounds are more felt than seen. Lucy Blackman calls this phenomenon 'sound-feeling'[13].

Often the skin sensation comes from sounds other people cannot hear. But there are no strict rules as the experiences, interpretations and responses change at different times. Some can be even *hit* by sounds. What is even more interesting, the sound can be both felt on their skin and seen by their eyes simultaneously. Too much noise creates visual chaos – making it impossible to interpret their environment and comprehend what is going on around them.

One of my earliest experiences of synaesthesia was during my teaching days at my school for autistic children. I brought some coloured alphabet blocks into the classroom for fun learning. But seven-year-old Lena definitely didn't think this idea was much fun. She grabbed a block and threw it across the room: "The colour is wrong! "C" isn't yellow, it's brown!"

Synaesthesia can indeed involve letters, words or numbers being experienced as colours. Sometimes numbers are experienced as shapes or forms. In the fascinating book *Born on a Blue Day*, autistic mathematician Daniel Tammet[14] describes experiencing numbers as cities which he can walk through.

There are still more puzzling variations: when abstract concepts such as, for example, units of time or mathematical operations, are perceived as shapes or colours (*conceptual synaesthesia*). So the answer to 6 + 2 may be 'green' (for 8)!

Synaesthetic experiences are involuntary; they are not just in the head, they are projected into the environment: individuals with synaesthesia actually see sounds, hear colours, etc. Interestingly, synaesthetic experience is very individual; for example, among people who see coloured sounds there is no specific colour for each sound from person to person.

One of the most common features of synaesthetes is their superior memory (due to their parallel sensations). They remember conversations, verbal instructions and spatial location of objects in every detail.However, this phenomenal experience, though very useful in remembering things, could lead to complications. Their understanding of spoken or written speech is literal. Each word evokes images that distracts them from the meaning of the sentenceas a whole.

Synaesthetes are observed to have uneven cognitive skills. They are reported to prefer order, neatness, symmetry and balance. They are more prone to unusual experiences such as déjà vu, clairvoyance, etc. Among their deficiencies, the most commonly reported are: right-left confusion, poor math skills and a poor sense of direction. Here we can see some similarity between the synaesthetic and autistic features.

This mysterious condition is not easily detected because many autistic children with synaesthesia don't realise that other people cannot, say, hear sounds while seeing colours. To them, it's a normal way to perceive the world. Even very articulate adults with autism find it difficult to express their experiences because they are so different from the 'norm'. And of course, unappreciated... (For many, though, synaesthesia can be a distinct advantage. The artist Kadinsky and some other artists, composers and writers have (had) this condition and use it for creative purposes).

When Alyosha is in a state of sensory overload, his synaesthetic experiences aggravate his condition, which can lead to panic attacks and meltdowns. After one of these 'incidents' he tried to give his explanation of what had happened: "In the shop I heard black, then the word broke down into pieces and they entered my eyes. I became blind because everything was black." At the time, I was bewildered with this explanation, and placed his 'reports' into the category 'confusing'. However, in 2011, I came across the account by Brian King[15], a social worker who is on the autism spectrum himself, as well as father of three autistic children. King says that when he is listening to someone speak, he can see each word; words scroll through the air in front of him. If someone repeats a word in a conversation, Brian sees it in a darker colour; and if his communicative partner emphasizes that word while speaking, it literally jumps out at him in 3D.

Alyosha sees not only colours in response to sounds, but also words when he hears them. If he sees the 'wrong word' (or as he says his 'eyes see the wrong word') we are all in trouble. His panic attack is not far away, and the consequences may be unpredictable.

* * * * *

Notes in the Margin –
Synaethesia

Synaesthesia is believed to be genetic. Most synaethetes don't complain of their condition because for them it is their normal perception of the world and they are not aware of it causing any disadvantages. Moreover, they often enjoy the colours of voices and emotions, tactile experience of music, smells of sounds and many other unique perceptions, and think that losing their unique perception would be upsetting, like 'losing one of the senses'.

However, it is true only if synaesthesia is unidirectional, whereas in case of 'two-way' (bidirectional) synaesthesia (when, for instance, a synaesthete not only sees colours when he hears sounds, but also hears sounds whenever he sees colours), the individual really suffers fromthe condition and can experience stress, dizziness and information overload. Because of this, they may avoid noisy or colourful places, and may withdraw completely. And if the synaesthete has autism (with other sensory problems as well) it becomes harder to deal with sensory overload.

A child can also experience problems with the voice of his/her communicative partner because the voice hurts or sends flashes of colour that disrupts the understanding. Or the voice may be so pleasant (with pleasurable sensory experiences – colour, movement, tactile sensations, odours) and fascinating that the child cannot focus on the conversation and lose the meaning of verbal utterances. In some situations, when somebody says something, a child might see the word, but if more people are talking in the same room, blurs appear that break the word, making comprehension difficult.

There's always a BUT – There are problems but it's a unique (and valid) way to perceive the world

Yes, sometimes there are problems, but a synaesthetic experience of each autistic person with synaesthesia is a unique (and valid) way to perceive the world they live in. Yes, it's puzzling for many others, but they must be puzzled as well – why can't other people see the range of colours in a noisy environment and the words floating in-between them?

It's useful to see synaesthesia as a distinct cognitive style. Seeing sounds/words/numbers in colours or feeling them as textures helps them to remember information. Often their secondary perceptions are much more vivid and vibrant than the primary ones so they provide additional cues to retrieve the information from memory. The combination of sensory imagery and a verbal thinking style provide original ways to solve problems.

Do's and Dont's – How to recognise synaethesia:

These are just a few indicators of possibility of synaesthesia.

Sensory synaesthesia:

Watch the reactions of the child to sensory stimuli: you can suspect synaesthesia if the child:

- covers/rubs/hits/blinks eyes in response to a sound/taste/smell/touch;
- covers/hits ears in response to a visual stimulus/taste/smell/touch/texture;
- complains about (is frustrated with) a sound in response to colours/textures/scent/flavour/touch;
- makes swallow movements in response to a visual/auditory stimulus/smell/touch;
- complains about (is frustrated with) taste in response to a visual/auditory stimulus/smell touch;
- covers/rubs/hits, etc. the nose in response to a visual/auditory stimulus/taste/touch;
- complains about (is frustrated with) feeling colours/sounds, etc. while being touched;
- complains about (is frustrated with) feeling being touched when being looked at;
- complains about (is frustrated with) backache/heat or cold in colourful/crowded/noisy place with lots of movement;
- involuntary movements/postures of the body in response to a visual/auditory stimulus/smell/taste.

Conceptual synaesthesia:

- complains about (is frustrated with) the 'wrong' colours of letters/numbers, etc. written on coloured blocks, etc.
- talks about 'wrong words', etc.;
- (when asked where he sees words, numbers, etc.,) points in the air in front of him.

There are many more unique experiences and interpretations of the environments which are hard to categorise as each individual develops his/her own systems and associations.

Some autistic individuals with synaesthesia can be intrigued by the colour and movement of the voice that they are unable to comprehend what the voice is saying and become confused and disoriented in social situations. If you suspect this is the case, talk in small 'doses' (1-2 sentences) and regularly pause to check if the child is 'with you' (following what you are talking about).

'Two-way' synaesthesia can be overwhelming, resulting in sensory information overload, stress and disorientation – making it impossible to interpret their environment and comprehend what is going around them. If this is the case, it's better to avoid noisy crowded places and/or provide respite from difficult situations. We should remember that the child's synaesthesia can be aggravated by many other sensory problems that can (and must) be addressed.

Some synaesthetes have only one form of synaesthesia, while others have several forms or variants of it. There are many forms of synaesthesia, which we don't know about yet. Listen to your child, don't dismiss their attempts to explain what they experience.

Pause for Thought – The Intense World Syndrome

Markram and colleagues[16] define autism as 'the intense world syndrome', where the core neurological pathology is excessive neuronal information processing and storage in local circuits of the brain, which gives rise to hyperfunctioning of the most affected brain regions. Autistic people perceive, feel and remember too much.

I prefer the metaphor of Parallel Sensory Perceptual Worlds: Though autistic people live in the same physical world and deal with the same 'raw material', their perceptual world turns out to be strikingly different from that of people without ASDs. All these experiences are based on real experiences, like those of people without autism, but these experiences may look, sound or feel different, or they may be interpreted differently. We think about the world in a way we experience it and perceive it to be. Different experiences bring different knowledge about the world. So how can we be sure that we are moving in the same perceptual/social world if our reconstructions of it are so different? How can we know that only our 'perceptual version' of the world is correct and theirs is wrong? Whatever the answers to these questions are, it is worth remembering that people with autistic conditions cannot help seeing and hearing the 'wrong thing', and they do not even know that they see or hear the 'wrong thing'. What we consider 'normal' connections between things and events do not make sense for them, and may be overwhelming, confusing and scary. In autism, any of the senses (or a combination of the senses) can be affected, bringing differences in interpretation and conceptualization of the environment they live in. In order to live in the same perceptual world (and to move in the same direction) we have to learn to switch from 'our' perspective to theirs. For example: Which way are the stairs headed?

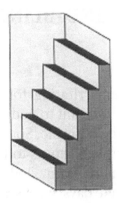

Up or down?

You cannot see both directions simultaneously and have to 'switch' your perception to observe each one. Those who live/work with autistic individuals have to learn to switch perspectives and imagine what's the world is like from the child's perspective, in order to join the child 'on his/her territory. Always try to imagine how the child sees, hears and feels. the world. Then consider what you can do to help the child to identify the 'right pieces of the jigsaw' and put them in the right places to get a clear picture of his/her environment. The difficulty of this exercise lies in our 'normal' sensory functioning.

12

THEORIES OF DIFFERENT MINDS: WHO IS MIND-BLIND?

One of my (often irritating for those around me) characteristics is, I want to understand anything and everything I encounter in my life. Sometimes it takes just a few minutes or a couple of hours to find the explanation to whatever it is that I am puzzled by at the time, but other times it might take days, weeks, months or years (and it continues now). Since my son's diagnosis, autism has become my obsession. From the very beginning, I started seeking answers to hundreds of questions, explanations of what was going on and why. Bullet-points books ('do this'/don't do this') were never good enough: if I didn't know WHY I had to do (or not to do) something, how could I implement this or that strategy to my son? I tried to find clues in the theories attempting to account for autism. However, every answer I found led to more questions.

I remember the first time I read about the lack of Theory of Mind in autism in the paper by Baron-Cohen and colleagues[17]. My reaction to the article was 'yes, but...', with the conclusion that the concept was one-sided. This is what I thought:

1.

Theory of Mind (ToM)* is defined as the ability to perceive the mental states of others; in other words, if autistic children lack ToM, it means they don't understand what other people are thinking, feeling and intending to do in different situations. In extreme cases (the originators of ToM claim) autistic children may have no concept of mind at all. New terms have been coined that have spread rapidly in the field – 'mind-blindness' and 'mind-reading'. This theory seems to explain a lot in 'autistic behaviours'.

Yes, but...

Yes, autistic children lack ToM and are 'mind-blind' to the thoughts, feelings and intentions of those around them. Non-autistic people's behaviours become unpredictable and confusing to an individual with autism.

But: Are non-autistic people 'mind-sighted' when they deal with persons with autism? Do they easily recognise feelings and intentions of individuals with autism? Considering that autistic and non-autistic people do *not share* sensory perceptual experiences due to differences in perceptual and cognitive functioning, don't non-autistic people find it difficult to take autistic individuals' perspectives? If autistic people lack Theory of Mind, then non-autistic individuals are sure to have deficits in the ability to understand the Theory of Autistic Mind. If we could remove one-sidedness from our interpretation of 'mind-blindness', we would see how limited we all are in our ability to 'mind-read'.

2.

The ToM is said to develop by the age of four.

Yes, but...

Yes, babies are not born with a 'ready-made' Theory of Mind. They develop it usually by the age of four. As their sensory experiences and thought-processes are similar to those around them, they soon become very successful in 'reading minds'.

But: Is the development of ToM spontaneous and independent from other variables (such as, for instance, differences in sensory experiences)?

For example, when Mother attempted to hug her little boy (expressing affection and happiness), instead of sharing the feeling of happiness and being loved (thus developing a 'normal ToM'), her son burst in tears because he couldn't tolerate being touched. Would he learn that mummy's smile and embrace mean 'affection'?

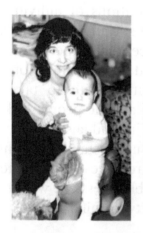
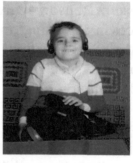

Or take another example, when Mother sent her son to his room to show her displeasure with his behaviour, would the boy who was overloaded with noise and movements of people around him and who suddenly found himself in the safety of his quiet room learn that it was supposed to be a 'punishment'?

Autistic individuals may learn to 'read (non-autistic) minds' later in life, using qualitatively different cognitive strategies and mechanisms. As a result, they are not quite successful in applying this theory in every-day life, with rapidly changing social situations, where they have to analyse each change as it comes. However, they are very skilful in Theory of Autistic Mind (ToAM).

3.
Numerous tests have been developed (the most famous one being the 'Sally and Ann test'*) that show that, unlike normally developing children and children with other developmental disabilities, autistic individuals cannot understand and predict actions of others.

Yes, but...

Yes, 'Sally & Ann' and other tests are widely used with autistic individuals (to prove they are 'mind-blind'?)
But: Why are there no tests to check *our* 'autistic mind-sight[18]

4.
The lack of ToM theory is very useful when applied to practical work with autistic people.

Yes, but...

139

Yes, it gives professionals and parents explanations of what otherwise have been seen as idiosyncratic behaviours, and provides ideas on how to address these problems. So-called lack of ToM in autistic children implies a different interpretation of 'rudeness' and 'deliberate stubbornness', as well as suggesting the necessity to explain explicitly our intentions and emotions to them.

But: Isn't it time we learn Theory of Autistic Minds that will help us understand our children better?

* * * * *

Notes in the Margin – Autism-unfriendly environment

Autistic children have to live in the world, which is not designed for them and they have to deal with people who, while being aware of the difficulties they experience, often overlook the efforts they make trying to survive in their (autism-unfriendly) environment. Our behaviour may seem equally 'bizarre' to autistic people. For example, how could one enjoy disco noises and strobe lights that are (as my son says) so prickly? For me, it was easy to sympathise with my son and other autistic individuals I was in contact with because I've experienced sensory sensitivities and filtering problems all my life. (Paradoxically, they become worse in old age. After being 'out there' for half a day, I need at least 8-10 hours of complete isolation (sort of sensory deprivation – no bright lights, no sounds, no movements, no people around). After that, I am able to face the public again. The problems start when it's impossible to find a place where I feel protected from sensory assaults, for example, on flights (when the passenger next to me was listening to music on his iPod– the headphones he was wearing didn't stop the intolerable noise that echoed in my head).

 ## There's always a BUT – More Theories of Mind

The ToM as a theoretical construct may be very useful not only when dealing with autistic and non-autistic populations, but also with different groups of people closely involved personally or professionally. Do professionals working with autistic children (and coming home free from autism) understand emotions and behaviours of the parents living with autism 24/7? On the other hand: Do parents who want the best for their autistic child understand professionals who have hundreds of autistic children in their files but limited resources? The answer to both questions is 'No'. It means the professionals lack Theory of Parents' Mind, while the parents lack Theory of Professionals' Mind. The logical solution would be to learn these different Theories of Mind and find the way to work together in order to create the world which would be comfortable to everyone concerned.

Do's and Dont's – 'Golden Rules' and Other Suggestions

Why? What? How? – Making sense of sensory needs:

Before considering 'what to do?' and 'how to do it?' we have to understand 'why?' (autistic children behave the way they do).

As we experience the world (through our senses) differently, our interpretation of 'autistic behaviours' (rocking, touching objects, etc., – often described as meaningless) is likely to be wrong. Even if we imitate them – our experiences will be different (for instance, by closing our eyes we won't recreate the experiences of the blind). 'Autistic behaviours' are often their (involuntary) attempts to organise and regulate sensory processing in order to make sense of the environment or to reduce painful experiences.

When we say that autistic children can be 'aggressive', we often forget that the real aggression comes from the 'normal' world – our highly sensitive children are hit by sounds and lights; tortured by textures and smells and experience other sensory assaults that we are so rarely aware of.

The main thing to remember is, their reactions and actions are logical and rational because they are dictated by their realities which are very different from a 'normal reality'.

Our intervention(s) (often based on the wrong assumptions) such as, for example, to reduce stimming* won't be beneficial for the child. Addressing 'problematic behaviours' (in order to eliminate them) by manipulating variables (ABA*) are not helpful (or are even harmful).

The focus should be on understanding the way they experience the world (and themselves), and interpret it from their perspective (ToAM), which may be very different from ours. So before you start teaching autistic children – learn about the way they perceive the world and themselves.

No two autistic individuals have exactly the same sensory perceptual profile, so each child's sensory needs are very specific.

To make necessary accommodations to the environment, we should know each child's particular difficulties. We have to identify and address the problems by:
-    either following the child's lead (if appropriate), or introducing different coping strategies and 'sensory aids'
-    desensitising the child (using 'sensory techniques' and therapies)

Work with autism – not against it

In order to survive in the world bombarding them with extraneous information, autistic children develop (voluntarily or involuntarily) the ability to control their awareness of incoming sensory stimuli to avoid sensory overload. Respect the children's efforts to protect themselves and to get meaning of what is happening around them.

If they avoid eye contact (to avoid overload/ hypersensitivity and to understand what's going on / is being said), follow their lead; for example, don't say, 'Look at me!' but rather sit next to your child and talk about what is in front of both of you.

Establish:
-    the most reliable sense for the child. It will help us to 'see' the environment from the child's point of view and 'speak' the same language
-    the most unreliable channel(s) and ways the child copes with the problem(s) (the child's coping strategies)

It is important to let the individuals use the sensory modality they prefer to check their perception. With appropriate support and treatment, they will learn to rely on other sensory channels.

Adjust the way you interact with the child: autistic children learn better with concrete information, whether it is visual, auditory, tactile, etc.
Let them use their ways to explore the world. In many ways 'autistic perception' is superior to that of non-autistics. Autistic individuals with their heightened senses often can appreciate colours, sounds, textures, smells, tastes to a much higher degree than people around them. Their gifts and talents should be nurtured and not ridiculed, as is often the case.

And remember, ALL autistic individuals (including so-called 'low-functioning') are highly (autistically) intelligent. That's how Jasmine O'Neill and Donna Williams put it:

"[Non-autistics] can be considered idiots in the autistic world[19]" and "appear to be thoroughly 'subnormal' by 'autistic' standards[20]".

And one more thing: Sometimes you will make mistakes. It's normal. Don't blame yourself. Learn from your mistakes.

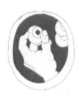 ## Pause for Thought – Learning About Theories of Different Minds (Tests & Activities)

Children's drawings often illustrate the way they perceive their surroundings and us. Two of my favourites are portraits of mothers created by two autistic boys with autism: D. and my son. Sometimes we call autistic children 'Martians' or extra-terrestrials, but don't we look like extra-terrestrials to them?

After one of the full-day trainings on sensory perceptual issues in autism (where we talked about the differences (both positive and negative ones) of sensory perception in autism, I challenged the participants (parents and professionals) to a simple activity: 'Think about the child you live/work with, then look at your reflection in the mirror but *through the eyes of this child*. Draw your portrait the way your child would[21].' I collected all the drawings and instructed them to ask the child to draw their portraits at home. The children's pictures they brought the next morning were compared to their versions. The results were very interesting.

For example:

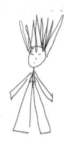

Mother's 'self-portrait'

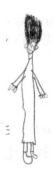

Her child'–S. with AS, 8 years old drawing 'Mother'

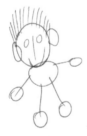

Mother's 'self-portrait'

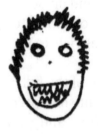

Her child's –A. with autism, 9 years old.

There are many tests to check whether autistic children have (or lack) ToM and plenty of books teaching autistic children to mind-read. But why don't we have ToAM tests? (With a few exceptionsxvi. Here are two (based on real life) stories for you to try:

Theory of Autistic Mind tests[1]

1. It's always been hard to buy presents for Nick (a 6-year-old non-verbal autistic boy) because one can't be sure what he really likes or wants. But once (just before Christmas) his mother was certain that the red toy car they saw in the shop was the gift he'd appreciate: Nick was fascinated with the toy – staring at it for what seemed an eternity, then took it from the shelf and gently touched the roof, and then the wheels. The next day Mother rushed to the shop to buy it. Back home, she wrapped it up and put it under the tree – anticipating the delight of her son on Christmas day. However, when Nick unwrapped his present, he started crying and pushed the toy away. The boy was inconsolable, and the day was ruined.

How would you interpret Nick's behaviour?
a) The boy didn't like the toy.
b) The boy liked the toy but expected something else.
c) The boy was shocked.

2. The mother is crying, her autistic son is standing in front of her, laughing loudly. How would you interpret the child's behaviour?
a) The child is happy
b) The child is upset
c) The child is indifferent.

However, as autistic children are very different in their sensory perception, there can be many other possible explanations:

[1] The answers are at the end of this chapter

Laughing is not always a laughing matter.
In autism, there is laughing/giggling and 'laughing/giggling'. There can be numerous reasons to laugh, which are difficult to understand by 'outsiders':

- Of course, autistic individuals laugh when they are happy, or if they find something funny.
- However, they often laugh to release fear, tension and anxiety.
Some with hypotactility/ hypoproprioception/ hypointeroception – either permanent or temporary) may laugh when they experience pain. For example, if the child doesn't feel anything, he can scratch himself, bite himself, bang his head against the wall – causing himself pain, to ease emptiness/ feel something; then even pain can be a pleasurable experience – it brings the feeling of being alive.
- They perceive certain (visual/auditory/tactile, etc.) stimuli differently: some of them can look/sound/feel funny – so the child can start laughing.
- Synaesthetic experiences often cause laughter: certain sounds, for example, can produce funny tickling on the skin or fascinating colours or sparkling lights and the air becomes full of light tongues of different colours.
- Funny memories triggered by something bring bursts of giggling. (While remembering, they re-experience those funny moments).

- To please others: when others are laughing at a joke or a funny situation, the child may start laughing as well (even without understanding of what's so funny). Seeing that his mother, for instance, was pleased with this reaction, next time in a seemingly similar situation, the child might start giggling to please those around him.

Theories of Parents' & Professionals' Mind

Parents living with their autistic children and professionals working with them experience their lives very differently. It's vital that both sides work together, always trying to understand Theories of Mind of their 'opponent'. (There are examples of tests for parents and professionals in *Theory of Mind and the Triad of Perspectives on Autism and Asperger syndrome*[22])

Just a few things to think about:

Professionals:
- If you don't like (or can't cope with) your job, you can quit any time. Most parents can't (and won't!) do that.
- Work together with parents. Each parent knows their child (and the child's autism) better than any expert. Let the parents be the interpreters of their child.
- Listen to the parents' concerns. If you think they are wrong, don't just dismiss their views. Remember, the parents are developing, too. Help them with the information and practical advice.

Parents:
- Never lie to your child. For instance, if you know it's going to hurt (for instance, a jab), say so but explain why it's

149

necessary and reassure that it'll be quick. You can reason with the child (even a non-verbal one).

- Create a description of your child (what you want the teacher to know about him) with bullet points, including what's he good at, what he struggles with, do's and don'ts, for example, "He likes to learn but finds it hard to sit quietly; - don't approach him directly; - sit next to him, not in front of him, etc." Keep it short. Teachers are busy, if reports are very long, they can skip and miss a lot of useful information about your child.

- Ask questions – to better understand how autism affects your child, what treatments and services are available. Knowledge is power.

Knowledge about autism (and definition of autism) is constantly changing. What is more, what was right yesterday, can become wrong (and harmful) today. Theories "explaining the enigma of autism" come and go but the child is growing and needs our help HERE and NOW.

The end?

– No! Far from it. Learning about autism never stops. (From my own experience, the more I learn about autism, the more I realise how little I know).

Knowledge about sensory perceptual differences is the basis for learning about (and establishing) communication with the child.

Answers to the ToAM tests:

1. *Answer*: c. – anything unpredictable will upset the child, even if it's something he really likes. Many autistic children don't like (even pleasant)

surprises. By the way, the following year Mother took the boy to choose his present. Back home, they wrapped it up together, and Nick put it under the tree himself. It was a delight to watch him unwrapping his present on Christmas day!

2. In this situation the right *answer* is *b*: The child is frightened because he doesn't understand what is going on and doesn't know what to do in this situation. Laughing/giggling is often caused by frustration and confusion.

GLOSSARY

A BA (Applied Behaviour Analysis) – focuses mainly on early intervention (pre-school years). The underlying principles are based on Skinnerian operant conditioning and behavioural discrete trials. The methods involve time-intensive, highly-structured, repetitive drills in which a child is given a command and rewarded each time he responds correctly. Challenging behaviours are addressed by using such strategies as ignoring, time out and shaping. (Thus, the ABA approach is primarily aimed at behaviours rather than the causes of the behaviours. What the ABA treatment does not take into account is that many different causes may produce the same 'behavioural picture'.) Behavioural discrete trial programmes start with achieving general compliance – training to get the child to sit in a chair, make eye contact and imitate non-verbal behaviour in response to verbal commands. Speech is taught as a verbal behaviour via verbal imitation, following one-step commands, receptive discrimination of objects, pictures, etc., and expressive labelling in response to questions.

Auditory Integration Therapy/Training (AIT) – The principle of AIT originated from the concept of the possibility of a cure by mechanical means. E.g., if the movement of a limb is restricted, it can be cured (trained) by special physical exercises to increase its mobility. The 'mechanical' treatment influences not only the related muscles but also the related area of the brain. AIT is aimed at 'retraining' the ear to reduce hypersensitivity to sounds. There are two main types of AIT: the Tomatis method and the Berard AIT. The AIT procedure involves:

·   audiometric testing to find out whether the person has 'auditory peaks' that can be reduced or eliminated by AIT

·   the filtering out of sounds at certain selected frequencies in accordance with the individual audiogram; where an accurate audiogram cannot be obtained, the basic modulation system without specific filters is used

·   the modulation of the music by alternatively dampening and enhancing, on a random basis, the bass and treble musical output; each session lasts 30 minutes, two sessions a day for ten days

·   another assessment of the person's hearing after five days to find out whether the auditory peaks are still present and whether there is a need to readjust filters. If the person has speech or language problems, after half the sessions the volume level for the left ear is reduced to stimulate the language development in the left hemisphere.

Candida albicans – a species of yeast (a single-celled fungus) that commonly lives in or on our bodies. It can be found on the skin, in the gastrointestinal tract, the mouth and the vagina. Most of the time, Candida albicans does not cause any problems. It even plays a part in digestion and absorption of nutrition. However, in some cases, Candida albicans becomes infectious when there is some change in the body environment that allows it to multiply out of control.

Echoemotica – the term coined by Stephen Shore to describe the phenomenon of taking on other person's emotion without realising that it's not yours.

Exposure therapy was originally designed to treat fear, anxiety (resulting in phobias). The general principle of the therapy is to gradually re-introduce a disturbing stimulus at progressively closer ranges until habituation occurs.

Genotype – the genetic constitution of an individual organism (often contrasted with phenotype)/the particular type and arrangement of genes that each organism has.

Gestalt – a shape, pattern or structure that, as an object of perception, forms a specific whole and has properties that cannot be completely deduced from knowledge of the properties of its parts. The term was originally used by a school of psychology – Gestalt psychology – which emphasises relational aspects, especially of perceiving in strong opposition to atomistic concepts.

Gestalt perception – the inability to distinguish between foreground and background information; perception of the whole scene as a single entity with all the details perceived (not processed!) simultaneously.

Gustation (the sense of taste) – the faculty of perceiving the sensation of a soluble substance in the mouth and throat. The receptors of taste are taste buds on the tongue, inside the cheeks, on the roof of the mouth and in the throat. There are between 2000 and 5000 taste buds that are subdivided into several categories of the primary tastes: sweet (near the tip of the tongue), salty and sour (on the sides of the tongue), bitter (on the back of the tongue) and spicy. The middle of the tongue, sometimes called the tongue's blind spot, has no taste buds. The tongue can also sense temperature and texture. The sense of taste is not very strong without the sense of taste.

Fading – decreasing the level of assistance needed to complete a task or activity.

Habituation – the diminishing of an innate response to a frequently repeated stimulus. It is a form of adaptive behaviour, a form of learning to stop responding to a stimulus which is no longer relevant.

Hearing – the faculty of perceiving sounds. The sense organs of hearing are the ears. The sound from each ear goes to the auditory cortex of the opposite brain hemisphere.

Heterogeneity – the quality or state of being diverse, different in kind; being different or opposite in structure, quality, etc. At present, there is a change of focus from the notion of the autism spectrum to heterogeneity, i.e., not autism but 'autisms'.

Holding therapy was originated by Martha Welch in the late 1980s and described as a 'miracle cure' for autism. The therapy is seen as strengthening the bonds of love between a mother and a child which are the foundation of happy and healthy development. It is assumed that when held safely in its mother's arms, the autistic child learns to overcome the fear of direct eye contact and close attachment. It was alleged that holding helps the child to release previously inhibited feelings of anger and rage. Despite the child's attempts to get free the mother holds the child firmly, supposedly giving the message that the mother's love is so strong that whatever the child does, whatever his/her feelings are, she can take care of him/her. Though it brought extreme distress and suffering to both the child and the parents who had to observe the suffering of the child they were trying to help (cure?), the parents were told this was the price they had to pay for a 'miracle'.

'Hug machine'/ 'Squeeze machine' – is a device consisting of two padded side-boards which are hinged near the bottom to form a V-shape. The person crawls inside and, by using a lever, provides the deep pressure stimulation. The lever operates an air cylinder, which pushes the sides together. The person can control the level of pressure he wants to stimulate.

Interoception – sensitivity to stimuli originating inside the body; perception of physiological feedback from the body. It is responsible for feeling of heart-beat, sickness, internal pain, thirst, hunger, bowel movement and other internal sensations.

Leaky gut syndrome – metabolic abnormalities like the incomplete breakdown of certain proteins, particularly, but not exclusively, gluten from wheat and casein from dairy products, that result in production of peptides which enter the bloodstream and cross the blood-brain barrier.

Minicolumns – these vertical columns are the smallest units of the brain capable of processing information

Olfaction (the sense of smell) – the faculty of perceiving odours or scents. It is the primary sensory channel in infancy. Olfactory receptors are located in the nostrils on the olfactory epithelium and deal with odour molecules in the air. There are about 10 million smell receptors in the nose, of at least 20 different types. Each type detects a different range of smell molecules. Smell plays an important role in the way we taste.

Perception – 1) the faculty of perceiving; 2) the ability of the mind to refer sensory information to an external object as its cause.

Phenotype – the set of the physical and biochemical characteristics of an individual resulting from the interaction of its genotype* with the environment.

Pica – craving for substances other than normal food (such as clay, soil, grass, hair) occurring as a symptom of a disease; a psychiatric / eating disorder characterised by the compulsive eating of non-food substances

Proprioception – the body awareness. The proprioceptive system (kinaesthetic sense) receives the information from contracting and stretching muscles, and the bending and compression of joints, and provides awareness of body position and posture of the body. Proprioceptors also identify the right amount of pressure to pick up something light or heavy.

Resonance – the term coined by Donna Williams to define the state when one 'loses oneself in' / 'becomes resonant with' something else. The person can merge with (lose oneself in) different sensory stimuli as if the person became part of the stimulus itself.

Sally and Ann test – one of the first ToM tests to check the ability to understand other person's perspective: the child sees a doll named Sally watch another doll named Ann place a marble into her basket. Ann leaves, and Sally moves the marble from the basket into her box. When Ann returns, the child is asked where Ann will look for her marble: in the basket or the box? Typically developing children and most children with Down syndrome will correctly infer that Ann will look in the basket because she doesn't know that the marble has been moved. Most children with autism will say that Sally will look where they, not Sally, saw her marble hidden.

Sensation – the consciousness of perceiving or seeming to perceive some state or condition of one's body or its parts or of the senses; an instance of such consciousness.

Sensory agnosia – an inability to process/interpret/recognise sensory information.

Stims, stimming – self-stimulatory or stereotypic behaviours: repetition of physical movements, hand-flapping, rocking, tapping things, spinning, repetition of sounds, words and phrases, etc.

Structure (of time/ place) – part of a structured teaching approach: structuring of the environment, time and activities to cue behaviour.

Tactility – the faculty of perceiving touch, pressure, pain and temperature. The sense of touch is one of the first senses to develop. The sense organ of tactility is skin. There are five different types of tactile receptors in the different skin layers: for light touch, pressure, pain, heat and cold.

Theory of Mind (ToM) – the ability to perceive the mental states of others. An inability to infer another mental state is termed *lack of Theory of Mind* or *mind-blindness*. In the 1990s, it was considered the central feature of autism.

Vestibular system – the sense organs of balance and gravity are located within the inner ear that detect movement and changes in the position of the head. The sense of balance is backed up by vision and by proprioceptors.

Vision – the faculty of seeing. The sense organs of vision are the eyes: they receive light and let it into the nerve ending (the sight receptors) at the back of the eyes (the retina).

1. Behavioural descriptions of autism in the two main classifications at the time – ICD-10 and DSM-IV – were based on Wing's Triad of Impairments: impairments of social interaction, communication, and stereotyped patterns of behaviour. It was only in May 2013, that the fifth edition (DSM-V) was published, which introduced considerable changes in the diagnostic criteria of ASD, including introduction of 'sensory symptoms' as essential for the diagnosis of autism.

2. Bogdashina, O. (2016): 2nd revised edition: Sensory Perceptual Issues in Autism: Different Sensory Experiences – Different Perceptual Worlds. London: Jessica Kingsley Publishers

3. Numerous individual differences, indicating possible subtypes based on different patterns of sensory perceptual problems have been reported, e.g.: Ausderau, K., Sideris, J., Furlong, M., Little, L.M., Bulluck, J., Baranek, G.T. (2013) National survey of sensory features in children with ASD: Factor structure of the Sensory Experiences Questionnaire (3.0).' Journal of Autism and Developmental Disorders 44, 4, 915-925;

Gonthier, C., Longuépée, L., Bouvard, M. (2016) 'Sensory processing in low-functioning adults with Autism Spectrum Disorder: Distinct sensory profiles and their relationships with behavioural dysfunction.' Journal of Autism and Developmental Disorders, 46, 9, 3078-3089.

Greenspan, S.I. and Wieder, S. (1997) 'Developmental patterns and outcomes in infants and children with disorders in relating and communicating: A chart review of 200 cases of children with autistic spectrum diagnoses.' Journal of Developmental and Learning Disorders, 1, 87-141.

4. There are more pronounced motor difficulties from adolescence into adulthood which impact on the ability to perform daily activities across the lifespan

5. Murchie, G. (1978) The Seven Mysteries of Life. Boston, MA: Houghton Mifflin.

6. Casanova, M.F., Buxhoeveden, D.P., Brown, C. (2002) 'Clinical and macroscopic correlates of minicolumnar pathology in autism.' Journal of Child Neurology, 17(9), 692-695

7. Williams, D. (1996) Autism: An Inside-Out Approach. London: Jessica Kingsley Publishers

8. Williams, D. (1996) Autism: An Inside-Out Approach. London: Jessica Kingsley Publishers

9. Koegel, R., Openden, D., Koegel, L. (2004) 'A systematic desensitization paradigm to treat hypersensitivity to auditory stimuli in children with autism in family contexts.' Research and Practice for Persons with Severe Disabilities, 29, 122-134.

10. Some professionals, trying to justify holding therapy, compare it with Temple Grandin's squeeze machine or describe it as a form of desensitisation. It couldn't be more far from the truth. The main difference is:

The squeeze machine and desensitisation do not imply force and allow the user to control the touch and pressure and to be able to stop the stimulation when it becomes too overwhelming or intense. Many autistic people are hypersensitive to tactile stimuli. Desensitisation technique presupposes gradual exposure to touch and pressure in a way which

is safe and enjoyable for a child.
Force holding has nothing to do with either these techniques or bonding with mother.

11. Williams, D. (1996) Autism: An Inside-Out Approach. London: Jessica Kingsley Publishers

12. Stehli, A. (1991) The Sound of a Miracle: A Child's Triumph Over Autism. New York: Avon Books.

13. Blackman, L. (2001) Lucy's Story: Autism and Other Adventures. London: Jessica Kingsley Publishers.

14. Tammet, D. (2006) Born on a Blue Day: A Memoir of Asperger's and an Extraordinary Mind. London: Hodder and Stoughton.

15. King, B.R. (2011) Strategies for Building Successful Relationships with People on the Autism Spectrum. London: Jessica Kingsley Publishers.

16. Markram, H., Rinaldi, T., Markram, K. (2007) 'The intense world syndrome – An alternative hypothesis for autism.' Frontiers of Neuroscience, 1. 77-96

17. Baron-Cohen, S., Leslie, A.M., Frith, U. (1985) 'Does the child with autism have a theory of mind: a case specific developmental delay?' Cognition, 21, 37-46.

18. See the first (though not scientifically validated) TOAM tests (to illustrate possible misunderstanding caused by lack of TOAM), Theories of Parents' and Professionals' Mind in Bogdashina, O. (2005) Theory of Mind and the Triad of Perspectives on Autism and Asperger Syndrome: A View from the Bridge. London: Jessica Kingsley Publishers.

19. Williams, D. (1998) .Autism and Sensing. London: Jessica Kingsley Publishers.

20. O'Neill, J. (1999) Through the Eyes of Aliens. London: Jessica Kingsley Publishers

21. A variant of this exercise is to draw the classroom from the child's perspective.
22. See the first (though not scientifically validated) TOAM tests (to illustrate possible misunderstanding caused by lack of TOAM), Theories of Parents' and Professionals' Mind in Bogdashina, O. (2005) Theory of Mind and the Triad of Perspectives on Autism and Asperger Syndrome: A View from the Bridge. London: Jessica Kingsley Publishers.

ABOUT THE AUTHOR

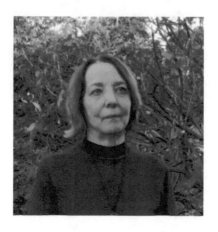

Olga Bogdashina, MA, MSc, Ph.D. is Co-founder of the International Autism Institute and Co-founder of the International Consortium of Autism Institutes. She has worked extensively in the field of autism as a teacher, lecturer and researcher. From 1994 till 2010, she's been Director of the first day centre for children with autism in Ukraine and President of the Autism Society of Ukraine 'From Despair to Hope'. She is Visiting Professor in Autism Studies at universities around the world, develops university (Autism Study) courses and training programmes for professionals and parents. Olga presents at national and international autism conferences and is an autism consultant for services for children and adults.

Olga lives in Yorkshire, UK. She has a son with classic autism (34) and a daughter (31).

To view more of her work and to follow her blog, visit her website - www.olgabogdashina.com

Olga's research interests are reflected in her books:

- Sensory perceptual Issues in Autism and Asperger Syndrome (2016). 2nd (revised) edition, London & New York: Jessica Kingsley Publishers;

- Communication Issues in Autism and Asperger Syndrome (2004). London & Philadelphia: Jessica Kingsley Publishers;

- Theory of Mind and the Triad of Perspectives on Autism and Asperger Syndrome (2005). London & Philadelphia: Jessica Kingsley Publishers;

- Autism and the Edges of the Known World: Sensitivities, Language and Constructed Reality (2010) London & Philadelphia: Jessica Kingsley Publishers.

- Autism and Spirituality: Psyche, Self and Spirit in People on the Autism Spectrum (2013). London & Philadelphia: Jessica Kingsley Publishers.

— • —

COMING SOON

This second book of the series *Autism: Becoming a Professional Parent* deals with cognitive, language and communication development in autism and provides ideas and tips how to help the child in which Olga shares what she's learned (and continue to learn) about autism.

This is especially aimed for 1) parents to guide them through the ins- and outs of not just living with – but flourishing – together with their autistic children and 2) professionals working with autistic population in order to help them understand autistic perspective and communication systems autistic individuals use.

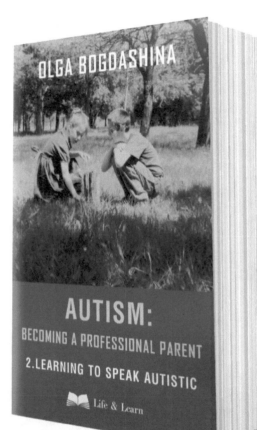

OLGA BOGDASHINA

AUTISM:
BECOMING A PROFESSIONAL PARENT
2.LEARNING TO SPEAK AUTISTIC

Life & Learn

Made in United States
Troutdale, OR
11/24/2023

14900363R00100